MIDWIFERY ESSENTIALS

Perinatal Mental Health

MIDWIFERY ESSENTIALS

Perinatal Mental Health

Michelle Anderson

RM, PG Cert HE., BSc Midwifery, BSc (Hons) Psychology
Senior Research Midwife
Royal Free London NHS Foundation Trust
Reproductive Health & Childbirth Research Champion
North Thames, United Kingdom

ELSEVIER

ELSEVIER

ISBN: 978-0-7020-8320-4

Content Strategist: Poppy Garraway
Content Development Specialist: Veronika Watkins
Publishing Services Manager: Deepthi Unni
Project Manager: Haritha Dharmarajan
Designer: Patrick Ferguson

Working together
to grow libraries in
developing countries

www.elsevier.com • www.bookaid.org

Printed in India

Last digit is the print number: 9 8 7 6 5 4 3 2 1

Contents

Michelle Anderson

Michelle Anderson

Contributors

Jane Anderson, BSc (Hons) Psychology, PG Diploma Psychodynamic Counselling, MBACP (accred.)
Women's Health Counsellor
Royal Free London NHS Foundation Trust

Michelle Anderson, RM, PG Cert HE, BSc Midwifery, BSc (Hons) Psychology
Senior Research Midwife
Royal Free London NHS Foundation Trust
Reproductive Health & Childbirth Research Champion
North Thames, United Kingdom

Cathy Ashwin, RN, RM, PGCHE, MSc, PhD
Freelance Midwifery Consultant; Honorary Assistant Professor
Academic Division of Midwifery
University of Nottingham
Nottingham, United Kingdom

Kate Clements, BSc (Hons), PG Cert
Named Midwife for Safeguarding
Maternity
Royal Free London NHS Foundation Trust
North Thames, United Kingdom

David Connor, Consultant Midwife, MSc, Advanced Practice Midwifery, BSc Midwifery, Diploma Adult Nursing
Head of Midwifery
University College London Hospital
London, United Kingdom

Judith Ellenbogen, MSc, CQSW, Diploma in Applied Social Studies, BA, MBACP (accred.)
Women's Health Counsellor
Obstetrics and Gynaecology
Royal Free London NHS Foundation Trust
North Thames, United Kingdom

Helen Griffiths-Haynes, RM, BSc (Hons), PGcert (Higher Education), LLM (Medical Law and Ethics)
Senior Lecturer in Midwifery
De Montfort University
Faculty of Health and Life Sciences
Leicester School of Nursing and Midwifery
Division of Maternal and Child Health
Leicester LE1 9BH

Sally Hines, PhD
Chair of Sociology
Sociological Studies
University of Sheffield
Sheffield, United Kingdom

Agnieszka Klimowicz, MD, PhD
Consultant Perinatal Psychiatrist
North London Partners
Specialist Perinatal Mental Health Service
North London, United Kingdom

Anna-Marie Madeley, RM, BSc (Hons) Midwifery, MSc, PG Cert, THE, FHEA Midwife
Lecturer and Doctoral Student
The Faculty of Wellbeing
Education and Language Studies
The Open University
Walton Hall, United Kingdom

Ruth Pearce, PhD, MA, BA (Hons)
Visiting Research Fellow
Department of Sociology
University of Surrey
Guildford, United Kingdom

Visiting Researcher
School of Sociology and Social Policy
University of Leeds
Leeds, United Kingdom

Research Coordinator
Trans Learning Partnership
United Kingdom

Carla A. Pfeffer, PhD
Associate Professor
Sociology
University of South Carolina
Columbia, SC, United States

Maureen Doretha Raynor, BEd, MA
Senior Lecturer (Midwifery)
School of Nursing and Midwifery
De Montfort University
Leicester, United Kingdom

Damien W. Riggs, PhD
College of Education, Psychology and Social Work
Flinders University
Adelaide, SA, Australia

Tania Staras, RM, BA, MA, PhD, PG Cert, FHEA
Principal Lecturer in Midwifery
School of Health Sciences
University of Brighton
Eastbourne, United Kingdom

Francis Ray White, PhD
Senior Lecturer in Sociology
University of Westminster
London, United Kingdom

Acknowledgements

As editor and co-author of this inaugural perinatal metal health book for midwives, there are a number of people I would like to acknowledge and thank.

Firstly, thank you to all the contributors and reviewers for sharing their knowledge and expertise. It is this which has enriched the text, bringing thought provoking and practical clinical scenarios to life.

Thank you to Alison Taylor, who supported the preliminary stages of this book and provided excellent feedback which helped shape the final version.

Thank you to Veronika Watkins for your help and support with content and chapters!

Thank you to Kate Clements for interesting discussions on perinatal mental health and content planning, which, again, helped to shape this book.

Thank you to Marcus and Millie for your words of encouragement.

Thank you to Michael for a consistent supply of coffee and chocolate.

Finally, thank you to all the midwives who take the time to read this book. I hope that by doing so, a greater understanding of perinatal mental illness will be achieved and that this newly acquired knowledge will be applied within the sphere and scope of midwifery practice.

Dedication

This book is dedicated to my daughter, Shanika, who lives with mental illness, but in her own words, is not defined by it.

Foreword

I am humbled and honoured to write the foreword for this brand new textbook, *Midwifery Essentials: Perinatal Mental Health*, having been first approached by the publisher to review the initial proposal a couple of years ago. I am convinced that this textbook, written by academics and clinical experts, will fill the significant void in the current body of textbook literature in this specific area of maternity care. It provides the depth and breadth of knowledge surrounding perinatal mental health and its application to practice, which will support students and registered health care professionals alike, in aspiring to deliver personalised, holistic and safe maternity care.

Mental illness affects men and women equally (World Health Organization [WHO], 2020). However, the disclosure of mental illness and the subsequent stigmatisation attached to the individual is known to impact on assessment, referral and subsequent initiation of timely care and treatment. In some cultures (explored in Chapter 5) to speak of mental health issues is considered a taboo subject often resulting in the individual being ostracised from their family and local community. It is vital that midwives and other health care professionals have an understanding of cross-cultural perspectives and socioeconomic status within the scope of perinatal mental health to support those who are often the most disadvantaged members of society, for example, refugees, asylum seekers, women prisoners and those from black, Asian and minority ethnic (BAME) and the lesbian, gay, bisexual, transgender and queer/questioning (LGBTQ plus) communities. The impact of language barriers and the role the partner plays in childbirth should also be considered as these can vary greatly globally.

Although years of underinvestment and neglect have affected the provision of mental health services, in recent years, the importance of the world's mental health has increasingly gained prominence within the media with high-profile individuals encouraging more openness in disclosure. It has been reported that in the United Kingdom alone, approximately 1:6 adults are likely to experience a common mental disorder such as anxiety or depression at some stage in their lives (Morris, 2019). As a consequence, mental illness represents the largest single cause of disability and related costs to the economy and in some instances may lead to maternal suicide (Knight et al., 2019). It is a certain therefore, that those reading this text, be it student midwives, registered midwives and other health care professionals with an interest in midwifery and maternity care, will at some point in their careers encounter women with mental illness or complex emotional needs.

Over the past 5 years, NHS England has extended its commitment to improving access to perinatal mental health services for a total of 66,000 women per year by 2024 (NHSE 2016, 2019). This includes strengthening multi-agency team working in continuity of carer teams, increasing perinatal mental health midwife specialists and physicians to ensure that all women with perinatal mental health issues receive the best possible care.

This textbook provides a comprehensive and systematic approach to perinatal mental health and contemporary midwifery practice through the range of chapters with a clear purpose to inform, inspire and provide a useful toolkit (found in Chapter 7), to assist midwives in supporting women with mental illness. It also offers advice on how midwives can take care of themselves and each other, acknowledging that mental health affects everyone. Case scenarios, summary boxes, examples of good practice and reflection points support the reader in developing a greater understanding of the content alongside being directed to additional sources such as further reading including web resources, useful contacts and training courses.

The first three chapters provide an overview focusing on describing primary mental health disorders and the pharmacological and non-pharmacological treatments used in pregnancy, including the risks and benefits to both mother and baby based on NICE (2014) recommendations. Psychological support, counselling and various therapies and techniques available to women with mental health issues are also explored.

The consequence of perinatal mental health is far-reaching and can have long-term effects not just for the woman and her partner but also her children in their emotional, social and cognitive development. Subsequent chapters discuss the parent–infant relationship in the context of perinatal mental health, recognising that partners may also experience anxiety and depression, although guidance on support for fathers remains limited. Chapter 8 shares the interesting findings from an original empirical research project on trans-pregnancy and sensitively explores how transgender people can experience isolation and gender dysphoria during pregnancy, highlighting that depression and suicide rates are higher within this community than in the general population. The chapter explores men, trans/masculine and non-binary peoples' experiences of childbirth, including the specific challenges that they face during pregnancy and makes useful recommendations for best practices for midwives working with this diverse population.

The book draws to a close by presenting the case as to how the facets of modern-day life, such as the COVID-19 pandemic and the explosion of digital and social media, may also impact on pregnancy and mental health. These are very pertinent issues that each and every one of us has a part to play in reviewing how our own practices may impact on the health (mental and physical) and wellbeing of others.

In my role as an educator and from a national and international context, I am keen to ensure that **all** midwives and health care professionals working in the field of maternity, women's and children's health are cognisant of how important **good** mental health is to the entire family across the globe. *Midwifery Essentials: Perinatal Mental Health* will go a long way in achieving this.

**Professor Jayne E Marshall, FRCM, PFHEA,
PhD, MA, PGCEA, ADM, RM, RGN**
Foundation Professor of Midwifery/Lead Midwife for Education
Interim Head of School of Allied Health Professions
School of Allied Health Professions
College of Life Sciences
George Davies Centre
University of Leicester
Leicester

Reference

Knight, M., Bunch, K., Tuffnell, D., & on behalf of MBRRACE-UK. (2019). *Saving lives, improving mothers' care – Lessons learned to inform maternity care from the UK and Ireland Confidential Enquiries into maternal deaths and Morbidity 2015–2017. Oxford: National Perinatal Epidemiology Unit, University of Oxford. Ireland Confidential Enquiries into Maternal Deaths and Morbidity 2015-17.* Oxford: National Perinatal Epidemiology Unit, University of Oxford.

Morris, M. (2019). *Mental health.* London: The Nuffield Trust.

National Institute for Health & Clinical Excellence (NICE). (2014). *Antenatal and postnatal mental health: Clinical management and service guidance. Clinical guideline [CG192].* London: NICE.

NHS England (NHSE). (2016). *The five year forward view for mental health. A report from the independent Mental Health Taskforce to the NHS in England.* London: NHSE.

NHS England (NHSE). (2019). The NHS Long Term Plan, London: NHSE.

World Health Organization (WHO). (2020). *Gender and women's mental health.* Retrieved January 2020 from https://www.who.int/mental_health/prevention/genderwomen/en/.

Perinatal Mental Health

Perinatal mental illness – It's not all in the mind

Michelle Anderson and David Connor

It was after my daughter was recovering from a period of mental illness that I began to think about how important it was for midwives to understand the complexities of mental health. Approximately one in six adults in the UK will experience a common mental disorder such as anxiety or depression (Morris, 2019). Mental health problems represent the largest single cause of disability in the UK and the cost to the economy is estimated at £105 billion a year (NHS England, 2016). Perhaps many of you reading this book will have personal experience of mental illness, whether it is yourself, a close family member or friend. Furthermore, I am almost certain that, as a midwife, at some point in your career, you will encounter women with mental illness or complex emotional needs. Therefore it is without question that mental health is equally as important as physical health.

It is worth noting that mental illness affects men and women equally; however, there are significant differences in the patterns of mental illness (WHO, 2020). For example, women are more likely to experience anxiety and depression (WHO, 2020). Women are also more likely to experience domestic abuse, which is a contributing factor to mental illness (WHO, 2020). There appears to be no gender difference in the incidence of mental health disorders such as schizophrenia and bipolar affective disorder, but women may experience *symptoms* of these illnesses differently (NIMH, 2020).

What is perinatal mental health?

Perinatal mental health specifically relates to the mental health of women during and after pregnancy. Women can develop mental health issues for the first time during pregnancy and after childbirth, so it is important for midwives to be mindful of this and to continually screen for changes to mental health throughout the antenatal and postnatal period.

Many women with existing mental illness will go on to have children. These include women with severe or complex mental illness; therefore it is imperative that midwives develop a good understanding of how to care for women presenting with various mental health conditions.

1

It is estimated that one in five mothers suffer from depression and anxiety in the antenatal period or in the first year after childbirth (NHS England, 2016). Furthermore, approximately one in 1000 women go on to develop postpartum psychosis and the risk increases if there is a history of mental illness in the woman or her immediate family (RCP, 2020). Suicide is the fifth most common cause of women's death during pregnancy and the postnatal period, but it is the leading cause of death in the first year after pregnancy (NDPH, 2018). About 6% of the women who died during pregnancy or in the year after giving birth in the UK between 2015 and 2017 had a mental health diagnosis or suffered from domestic or substance abuse (Marriott et al., 2019). The consequence of perinatal mental health is far reaching and can have long-term effects not just for the woman and her partner but also her children in their emotional, social and cognitive development (NHS England, 2020).

Partners of pregnant women may also be affected by mental illness and this can have an impact on the woman and the rest of the family. A report from the Royal College of Obstetricians and Gynaecologists (RCOG) found that many men experienced low mood or depression, followed by anxiety during or after pregnancy, but that support was lacking, as health professionals predominantly focused on the health of the mother and baby (RCOG, 2017). As midwives, we must strive to ensure that we acknowledge the mental health of partners as part of providing holistic care to the woman and her newborn baby.

Lesbian, gay, bisexual, transgender and queer/questioning (LGBTQ+) and black, Asian and minority ethnic (BAME) communities are more likely to experience suicidal thoughts and actually attempt suicide (MHFA, 2019). LGBTQ+ communities are also more likely to develop anxiety disorders, whereas psychosis is more common amongst BAME groups (MHFA, 2019). The recent MBRRACE report (2015–2017) states that there is a 5-fold difference in maternal mortality rates amongst women from black ethinc backgrounds and a 2-fold difference in women from Asian ethnic backgrounds compared to white women (MBRRACE, 2019). Although this is not solely due to mental health, the recognition that BAME communities are more likely to attempt suicide should not be ignored in light of these findings, especially as it is estimated that black and black British women are more likely to have a common mental health problem (29.3%) compared with white British women (20.9%), and non-British white women (15.6%) (McManus et al., 2016).

Consideration should also be given to gender identity. Gender identity describes whether individuals identify as a man, woman or many other genders (Obedin-Maliver & Makadon, 2016). A transgender person is someone whose gender identity is not congruent with the sex they were assigned at birth (Makadon et al., 2015). It has nothing to do with who they are emotionally, romantically or sexually attracted to but is instead how they choose to live and bring their physical body into alignment with internal gender identity (Obedin-Maliver & Makadon, 2016). Transgender individuals can experience isolation and gender dysphoria during pregnancy. It is important for midwives to be aware that depression and suicide rates are higher in transgender individuals than among the general population; therefore extra vigilance is required when screening for depression and anxiety during pregnancy and after childbirth for these individuals (Obedin-Maliver & Makadon, 2016).

Poverty and socioeconomic disadvantage is another contributing factor towards poor mental health; 29% of women in poverty are more likely to experience a common mental health condition compared with 16% of women not in poverty (The Woman's Mental Health Taskforce, 2018). Women who are asylum-seekers or prisoners may also feel isolated and experience poor mental health.

Navigating the twists and turns of mental health services

Some women do not access mental health support for fear of being judged on their ability as a parent, or at worst, having their child removed (The Woman's Mental Health Task Force, 2018). Many women worry about the social stigma attached to mental illness (MHF, 2020). It is important for the midwife to be aware that women may find it difficult to disclose worries about their mental health for fear of prejudice. Therefore the midwife should offer a safe space for the woman to talk about any health concerns, including mental health.

It is reported that BAME women face additional barriers to accessing mental health support and services. These include issues with recognising and accepting mental health problems, a reluctance to discuss psychological stress and seek help, a negative perception of mental health and worries about social stigma (The Woman's Mental Health Task Force, 2018).

The level of support given by mental health services can vary significantly. It is widely reported that NHS mental health services have faced years of underinvestment and neglect (Kings Fund, 2019). However, to actually experience the lack of resources available is fundamentally distressing. I speak from my daughter's experience and witnessing the disparity in care first hand, especially during periods of her being acutely unwell. At times, I can honestly say, there was no one to turn to in terms of support. Living with a severe mental health condition is complex and difficult enough without having to navigate a turbulent and underfunded health care system. However, the future is beginning to look hopeful with mental health services receiving the long-awaited attention and additional funding it so desperately requires (Kings Fund, 2019). Even so, there is still much work to be done.

The future of perinatal mental health services

NHS England's *Five Year Forward View for Mental Health* (2016) set out an agenda to reform mental health care, which included perinatal mental health (NHS England, 2016). A clear implementation plan was developed detailing the aims and objectives of a 5-year strategy which aimed to improve investment and access to mental health services by 2020–2021 (NHS England, 2016).

The aims included the following:

- Over 120,000 more people are expected to receive mental health care and treatment in priority services in 2016–2017.
- The Mental Health Investment Standard is planned to be met across England as a whole in 2017–2018 and 2018–2019.
- The first national access standards for mental health treatment have come into effect – with the waiting time targets met.
- A new Mental Health Dashboard has been launched to provide unprecedented transparency of performance against key indicators.
- The first comprehensive all-age mental health workforce strategy has been co-produced for publication in April 2017

  (*Taken from The Five Year Forward View for Mental Health: One Year On, 2017.*)

In terms of perinatal mental health, the *Five Year Forward View* proposed that specialist mental health services should be available for all women and their families who need them (NHS England, 2017). The Perinatal Specialist Development Fund was launched in August 2016, with £40 million available over a 3-year period to help expand and improve service in 20 areas across England, which included 90 clinical commissioning groups (CCGs) (NHS England, 2017). So far, the programme has been extremely successful with all areas of England now able to access specialist perinatal community teams and the number of inpatient mother and baby units risen from 15 to 19 (Marriott et al., 2019). However, there is still more work to do to ensure that all women who need perinatal mental health services have access to them. NHS England's *The Long Term Plan* (2019) is further committed to improve access to perinatal mental health services for a total of 66,000 women per year by 2023–2024 (Marriott et al., 2019).

Perinatal mental health and midwifery

Midwives now play a fundamental role in the care of women with perinatal mental illness. Better Births and the roll out of continuity of carer service models have contributed to increased support for women with perinatal mental health issues and the benefits of this are widely documented (see Chapter 7 for further details). The introduction of perinatal mental health midwives and midwifery specialist teams are important to ensure that all women with perinatal mental health issues receive the best possible care during the pregnancy continuum in collaboration with multi-disciplinary teams. Specialist mental health midwives are well placed to optimise care for women and their families who experience mental illness (RCM, 2018). However, the RCM (2018) report on specialist mental health midwives states the following:

> Specialist Mental Health Midwives play a crucial role in improving the quality of maternity services and supporting the development and implementation of integrated pathways of care for women with peri-natal mental illness. They are a critical part of multiagency perinatal mental health clinical pathways. However they are neither a substitute for specialist perinatal mental health care, nor for the mental health care delivered by all midwives. Mental health care is a core part of the role of all midwives: good maternity care means achieving good maternal mental and physical health, thereby improving outcomes for women and their families in this generation and the next.

Many midwives lack confidence when approaching women with mental health issues or those with complex social needs. This is generally because of poor or insufficient training, undocumented histories in maternal notes, poor continuity of care, lack of support services and reluctance from women to discuss their mental health issues (RCM, 2018).

One of the reasons for this book is to provide a comprehensive and systematic approach to perinatal mental health and midwifery practice. It is hoped that this resource will inform, inspire and provide a 'toolkit' to help midwives support women with mental illness. It also offers advice on how midwives can take care of themselves and each other, because mental health affects everyone. We are all human.

On a final note, I have experienced firsthand how difficult it is to watch a loved one go through an acute episode of severe mental illness and how the gaps in mental health services are very real. The toll this takes on the person suffering from the illness and the impact on family members should not be underestimated. So, as midwives, let us advocate for better mental health service provision and strive to support women and their families with kindness and understanding.

> *People will forget what you said, they will forget what you do but they will never forget how you made them feel.*
>
> ~Maya Angelou

References

Makadon, H. J., Mayer, K., & Potter, J. (2015). *Fenway guide to lesbian, gay, bisexual, and transgender health* (2nd ed.). Philadelphia: American College of Physicians [Google Scholar].

Marriott, S., Sleed, M., & Dalzell, K. (2019). *Implementing routine outcome monitoring in specialist perinatal mental health services*. Child Outcomes Research Consortium (CORC). Retrieved January 2020 from https://www.england.nhs.uk/wp-content/uploads/2019/12/Implementing-routine-outcome-monitoring-in-specialist-mental-health-services.pdf.

McManus, S., Bebbington, P., Jenkins, R., & Brugha, T. (Eds.). (2016). *Mental health and wellbeing in England: Adult Psychiatric Morbidity Survey 2014*. Leeds: NHS Digital.

Mental Health First Aid (MHFA) England. (2019). *Mental health statistics*. Retrieved January 2020 from https://mhfaengland.org/

Morris, J. (2019). *Mental health. The Nuffield Trust*. Retrieved January 2020 from https://www.nuffieldtrust.org.uk/news-item/mental-health-1

National Institute for Mental Health (NIHM). (2020). *Women and mental health*. Retrieved January 2020 from https://www.nimh.nih.gov/health/topics/women-and-mental-health/index.shtml

NHS England. (2016). *The five year forward view for mental health. A report from the independent Mental Health Taskforce to the NHS in England*. Retrieved January 2020 from https://www.england.nhs.uk/wp-content/uploads/2016/02/Mental-Health-Taskforce-FYFV-final.pdf

NHS England. (2017). *The five year forward view for mental health: One year on*. Retrieved January 2020 from https://www.england.nhs.uk/wp-content/uploads/2017/03/fyfv-mh-one-year-on.pdf

NHS England. (2019). *The NHS Long Term Plan*. Retrieved January 2020 from https://www.longtermplan.nhs.uk/wp-content/uploads/2019/08/nhs-long-term-plan-version-1.2.pdf

Nuffield Department of Population Health (NDPH). (2018). *New report on UK deaths during and after pregnancy*. Retrieved January 2020 from https://www.ndph.ox.ac.uk/news/new-report-on-uk-deaths-during-and-after-pregnancy

Obedin-Maliver, J., & Makadon, H. (2016). Transgender men and pregnancy. *Obstetric Medicine*, 9(1), 4–8. https://www.ncbi.nlm.nih.gov/pmc/articles/PMC4790470/#bibr28-1753495X15612658.

Royal College of Midwives. (2018). *Specialist mental health midwives. What they do and why they matter.* https://www.rcm.org.uk/media/2370/specialist-mental-health-midwives-what-they-do-and-why-they-matter.pdf

Royal College of Obstetricians and Gynaecologists. (2017). Maternal mental health – women's voices. RCOG. Retrieved January 2020 from https://www.rcog.org.uk/globalassets/documents/patients/information/maternalmental-healthwomens-voices.pdf

Royal College of Psychiatrists (RCP). (2020). *Postpartum psychosis.* Retrieved January 2020 from https://www.rcpsych.ac.uk/mental-health/problems-disorders/postpartum-psychosis

World Health Organization (WHO). (2020). *Gender and women's mental health.* Retrieved January 2020 from https://www.who.int/mental_health/prevention/genderwomen/en/

The Kings Fund. (2019). *Mental health: Our position.* Retrieved January 2020 from https://www.kingsfund.org.uk/projects/positions/mental-health

The Woman's Mental Health Taskforce. (2018). *Final report. Agenda* (Alliance for Women & Girls at Risk). Department of Health & Social Care. Retrieved January 2020 from https://assets.publishing.service.gov.uk/government/uploads/system/uploads/attachment_data/file/765821/The_Womens_Mental_Health_Taskforce_-_final_report1.pd

CHAPTER 1

An overview of perinatal mental health conditions

Agnieszka Klimowicz and Michelle Anderson

Identifying mental illness

Perinatal mental illness (PMI) affects up to 20% of women who are pregnant or have a baby under the age of 1 year (Public Health England Guidance, 2019). While PMI is common, many conditions remain under-detected and under-treated. Midwives play a significant role in the identification of mental health problems, alongside general practitioners (GPs) and health visitors. The importance of discussing mental wellbeing with women at the beginning of pregnancy and beyond should not be overlooked. Changes to mental health can be subtle and difficult to detect and may require the midwife to gently explore concerns that arise during the course of the pregnancy and postnatal period (as discussed further in Chapter 7). The aim of this chapter is to focus on describing primary mental health disorders as a general overview. It is recommended that further reading be undertaken to gain greater depth and understanding of each condition discussed.

Detection and prediction

The identification of mental health conditions consists of:

1. detection of the current symptoms and
2. prediction of the risk of the occurrence of mental health disorder (by taking personal and family history).

Diagnosis of functional (primary) mental health disorder is made after the exclusion of medical conditions or substance misuse. Changes in mental state (such as anxiety) can be induced by psychoactive substances, such as alcohol, cannabis, cocaine, stimulants, caffeine, hallucinogens, etc. Some medical conditions can cause secondary mental health problems; for example, hypothyroidism can cause depression, and anaemia can sometimes cause anxiety, low mood and tiredness.

The causality of mental disorders is unclear and likely multi-factorial (as discussed in other chapters); however, genetic and psychosocial factors will usually contribute. Many disorders first occur after significant life event(s) or are associated with psychosocial stressors, but symptoms may also appear without any apparent triggers.

Many symptoms of mental illness can be experienced naturally in a variety of situations. Therefore diagnosis is usually made on the basis of significant impairment in personal, family, social, educational, occupational or other important areas of day-to-day functioning. People with more complex mental health problems can have a number of psychiatric diagnoses (co-morbidities) as their symptoms do not easily fit into one category.

PMI can be pre-existing or new onset during the course of the pregnancy or postnatal period. Symptoms do not significantly differ in their *form* from those of the non-pregnant population; however, significant psychosocial changes, including the transition into motherhood, mean that *the content* of the symptoms will likely be focussed on the pregnancy and/ or the newborn. Additionally, the time of pregnancy and after birth gives rise to natural anxieties which in turn colour pre-existing or new-onset mental disorders with anxious feelings and preoccupations. The unique physiological state of pregnancy and hormonal changes around the time of birth and after can reveal biological vulnerability to changed mental state in a subgroup of women.

The incidence and prevalence of mild to moderate depression and anxiety are similar during pregnancy and the postpartum period. However, there is an increased incidence of severe non-psychotic depressive illness in the early weeks following birth. These conditions may initially present as anxiety and depression in the first 2–6 weeks following birth and can deteriorate rapidly.

The rate of new-onset serious mental illness is not elevated during pregnancy, but it can increase after birth. However, relapses of serious affective disorder (bipolar illness and severe depression) do occur during pregnancy, particularly if medication has been stopped. The majority of acute-onset serious perinatal disorders present as a psychiatric emergency in the days and weeks following childbirth.

More significant or complex mental health problems can affect parenting or be perceived as such. Pregnant women and those who have small children might be reluctant to seek help early due to the perceived stigma of mental illness. Some women may worry about how they will be judged as mothers by health professionals and/or have anxiety that their child(ren) will be taken away. Unfortunately, without treatment and support, even otherwise episodic mental health conditions can become chronic during pregnancy and the postnatal period. Recovery is often impeded by sleep deprivation and the increased responsibilities of new motherhood. It should be noted that adolescent women are more likely to face higher pregnancy-related maternal and perinatal morbidity and mortality than adult women

Box 1.1 Practice learning point

Depressive and anxiety *symptoms* occur in the majority of mental health illness and do not always constitute, *per se*, diagnosis of depression or anxiety – see, for example, the following clinical vignette:

Helen is 32 weeks pregnant with her second child and was referred by her midwife to the specialist perinatal mental health service with information that she experiences severe anxiety and has difficulty leaving her house. She has recently moved into the area and transferred her care from another hospital.

During psychiatric assessment, she revealed that she was diagnosed with schizophrenia a few years ago and takes olanzapine 20 mg daily (maximum BNF dose of antipsychotic medication; see Chapter 2 for further information on medication). Her husband recently left her, and she has become more paranoid, feeling safer in her home. She occasionally hears undifferentiated voices. She also suffers from diabetes.

Urgent perinatal mental health care/birth planning was subsequently arranged in collaboration with the wider multi-disciplinary team.

(World Health Organization (WHO), 2020). Although maternal mortality due to suicide in the United Kingdom is low, women are at much higher risk of suicide at this time of their lives that at any other. Suicide is the second largest cause of direct maternal deaths and it remains the leading cause of direct deaths occurring within a year after the end of pregnancy (Knight & MBRRACE, 2019) (as discussed in Chapter 8).

An overview of mental health conditions

The most common mental disorders are those of depression and anxiety.

Depression

Perinatal (antenatal and postnatal) depression is estimated to occur in 10%–15% of women in developed countries (Royal College of Psychiatrists (RCPsych), 2018). Approximately one-third to half of all affected women experience more severe depression (major depression). In pregnancy, depressive symptoms might be new-onset or relapse of a *depressive disorder* (Marcus, Flynn, Blow, & Barry, 2003; Shakeel et al., 2015). Depression usually has an *episodic course*, but chronic course is possible and called *dysthymia* (mild, chronic depression). Depressive episodes can be mild, moderate and severe.

Depression occurring in pregnancy can prevent bonding with the baby due to the reduction of positive feelings (Dubber, Reck, Muller, & Gawlik,

2014). Depression after birth can additionally interfere with forming a new identity as a mother, and often the woman will view motherhood as difficult (Leach, Marino, & Nikevic, 2019). It is worth noting that depressive episodes frequently co-occur with anxiety symptoms and even more so in pregnancy and after birth (Biaggi, Conroy, Pawlby, & Pariante, 2016). The risk of relapse in depressive illness can be as high as 50% (Sim, Lau, Sim, Sum, & Baldessarini, 2016); therefore it is important that the midwife screen for symptoms of depression throughout the course of the pregnancy.

Box 1.2 Symptoms of depression

- Low mood
- Low energy
- Lack of joy (anhedonia)
- Reduced self-esteem
- Feelings of guilt
- Pessimistic view about self, others and the future
- Feelings of hopelessness
- Indecisiveness, lack of motivation
- In more severe depression the following occur: insomnia, lack of appetite, speaking or moving more slowly than usual, low energy and ideas or acts of self-harm.
- Very severe depression can be accompanied by psychotic symptoms such as delusions and hallucinations.

Box 1.3 Practice learning point

- Depression is a highly recurring condition.
- If a person has a history of depressive episodes only, the disorder is called **unipolar depression**.
- If a person has a history of episodes of elated mood (mania or hypomania), depressive episode will be a part of **bipolar affective disorder (BAD)**, which is a severe mental illness with different risks in pregnancy and postpartum, requiring different treatment (see section on BAD at the end of this chapter).
- Bipolar and unipolar depression can appear similar. It is not usually possible to differentiate between them based only on the symptoms.
- Diagnosis can be changed from depressive disorder to BAD after an episode of elated mood. The postpartum period is associated with a small increased risk of transition to BAD.
- Depression is approximately two to three times more common in people with a chronic physical health problem than in people who have good physical health (NICE, 2009).

Baby blues

Baby blues is a transient period of increased mood lability in the first week after birth. Prevalence ranges from 26% to 84% in postpartum women (O'Hara & Wisner, 2014). Baby blues is associated with significant biological and psychological changes occurring a few days after birth.

Symptoms include dysphoric mood, crying, mood lability, anxiety, insomnia, loss of appetite and irritability (O'Hara & Wisner, 2014). It is *not* a mental disorder, and good sleep, practical help and reassurance will likely suffice for symptoms to resolve. However, baby blues might also be an early indicator of evolving postnatal mood disorder. Depression is diagnosed if the symptoms persist for most days in a 2-week period or are becoming worse and significant.

However:

- Significant insomnia and anxiety present early after birth and should not automatically be labelled as baby blues.
- Similarly, symptoms of baby blues or mild depression *before or after* birth, occurring in a woman with a history of significant depression or bipolar affective disorder (BAD), are predictors of relapse and should be treated accordingly.

Baby pinks

Little is known about this mood state, but it seems to occur early after birth and can affect approximately 1 in 10 women (Heron & Oyebode, 2011). The symptoms are similar to hypomania; for example, a new mother feels great and has increased energy levels. If the woman is able to sleep and rest adequately, this might not be a problem. However, baby pinks tend to occur more frequently in women with a history of mood disorder and might be a predictor of later occurring depression or psychosis (Heron, Craddock, & Jones, 2005). In particular, increased talkativeness, engaging in lots of tasks without their completion and reduced need for sleep require prompt attention from a mental health professional (Heron & Oyebode, 2011). Lack of sleep for a few days can give rise to bizarre ideas evolving into puerperal psychosis, which is a medical emergency. The mother should not be left with the baby unsupervised if any concerning behaviour or ideas are observed, and she should be referred for assessment by the mental health team operating in an acute setting.

Anxiety disorders

Anxiety disorders can affect up to 15% of pregnant women and about 8% after childbirth (O'Hara & Wisner, 2014).

Box 1.4 Practice learning points

Detection

NICE (2014) recommends asking the following questions about symptoms of depression as part of a general discussion about a woman's mental health and wellbeing:

- During the past month, have you often been bothered by feeling down, depressed or hopeless?
- During the past month, have you often been bothered by having little interest or pleasure in doing things?

Prediction

- Depression in pregnancy is one of the strongest predictors of depression postnatally.
- Women with a history of depression have a high chance of relapse during pregnancy and/or the postnatal period.
- A personal and family history of severe mental illness, particularly that of perinatal mental illness, should also be considered.

Anxiety is a normal feeling in certain situations, for example, before an examination or job interview. Anxiety becomes a clinical problem when it is overwhelming and/or constant. Anxiety disorders can have a chronic or remitting course. It is not unusual for a sufferer to have symptoms of a few anxiety disorders; for example, a person with general anxiety disorder (GAD) can develop panic disorder, or severe agoraphobia can result in panic attacks. Milder forms of anxiety disorders can be effectively treated with self-help or psychological therapies. Very severe or complex anxiety disorders might require pharmacological interventions (Table 1.1).

A significant sign of severe anxiety is avoidance. Avoidant behaviours take the edge off anxious thoughts or temporally eliminate them. However, avoidance can also reinforce anxiety. These behaviours can significantly limit day-to-day functioning.

Tokophobia

Tokophobia is a specific phobia where the woman experiences an extreme fear of pregnancy. It can lead to avoidance of childbirth. Worry about childbirth is common in pregnancy; however, tokophobia is very different and can be debilitating for the woman whereby her fears affect daily life. Tokophobia can be *primary* or *secondary*. *Primary tokophobia* is a morbid fear of childbirth in a woman who has had no previous experience of pregnancy. *Secondary tokophobia* usually develops after a traumatic or distressing birth (Hofberg & Brockington, 2000). Tokophobia can also be a symptom of depression or posttraumatic stress

Box 1.5 Screening for anxiety

Detection

NICE (2014) recommends screening for anxiety as part of a general discussion about a woman's mental health and wellbeing:

- Over the last 2 weeks, how often have you been bothered by feeling nervous, anxious or on edge?
- Over the last 2 weeks, how often have you been bothered by not being able to stop or control worrying?

Practice learning point

It is also useful to ask the following:

- Do you find yourself avoiding places or activities, and, if so, does this cause you problems?

Positive answers to the above one or more questions will require further exploratory discussion/assessment and, if required, a referral to the general practitioner or, if more significant mental health problems are suspected, to a mental health professional.

Note: New-onset, significant or deteriorating anxiety occurring suddenly towards the end of pregnancy and in early weeks after birth, in a woman without a longstanding history of anxiety disorder, requires further evaluation for more severe perinatal mental illness and will usually require a referral to (perinatal) mental health services.

---

disorder (PTSD) (Hofberg & Brockington, 2000). For some women, the fear of childbirth can be so severe that she avoids pregnancy, even if a child is desired.

Obsessive compulsive disorder

Obsessive compulsive disorder (OCD) is characterised by intrusive thoughts, images or urges (obsessions) and/or compulsive behaviours. OCD occurs in about 1% of the female population, 2% of women who are pregnant and closer to 2.5% of women postnatally, but the rate might be as high as 5% (O'Hara & Wisner, 2014). The relatively high prevalence suggests that pregnancy and childbirth might act as a trigger for OCD (Forray, Focseneanu, Pittman, McDougle, & Epperson, 2010).

Obsessions are unwanted (ego-dystonic), cause anxiety or unease and are usually a source of significant distress. The sufferer tries to ignore, suppress or control them with compulsive behaviours that give temporary relief (Table 1.2). For example, persistent thoughts that the gas on the cooker was not switched off after going to bed might lead to constantly checking the cooker throughout the night.

OCD in pregnancy and after birth might include worrying or intrusive thoughts about harming the baby, which can cause very significant distress to the mother. Mothers with intrusive worries about the health of their

Table 1.1: Types of anxiety disorders

General anxiety disorder (GAD) is the most common anxiety disorder. People with this fluctuating and chronic condition suffer from general apprehension ('free-floating anxiety') or excessive worries about multiple everyday events. They cannot relax, and they have variable physical symptoms such as shaking, excessive sweating, palpitations, tiredness, dizziness, epigastric discomfort, etc. GAD appears to be more common in women.

Panic disorder is when the most severe form of anxiety, *panic attack*, occurs. Panic attacks are usually very intensely felt with a plethora of physical symptoms, and the sufferer might develop a fear of being out of control or 'mad'. In between panic attacks, the sufferer develops persistent worries about having another panic attack (anticipatory fear or *'fear of fear'*). The latter might be more disabling than the actual panic attack.

Phobia is an overwhelming fear of an object, place, situation, feeling or animal. Phobia is diagnosed when the fear is exaggerated.

Specific phobia is, for example, fear of spiders, heights, closed spaces (*claustrophobia*) or bodily phobias such as blood, vomit or injections.

Agoraphobia is a type of complex phobia in which the sufferer is frightened in situations/places from which escape might be difficult or help not available (crowded places, supermarkets, public transportation, being outside, being home alone, etc). There is a fear of a particular negative outcome in such situations, for example, that of a panic attack or embarrassing physical symptoms.

Social anxiety disorder is fear in social situations, for example, during conversation or being observed while eating and drinking or performing in front of others (performance anxiety). The sufferer fears negative evaluation.

Hypochondria is fear about the possibility of having serious, progressive or life-threatening disease(s). The person misinterprets bodily signs or symptoms and might excessively seek professional attention but does not feel reassured after appropriate medical evaluations and investigations (WHO, 2020).

From World Health Organization (WHO). (2020). *ICD-11: Mental health*. https://www.who.int/health-topics/mental-health#tab=tab_1.

Box 1.6 Practice learning point

When a woman suffering from tokophobia and requests a caesarean section, NICE (2017) recommends a referral to a health care professional with expertise in providing perinatal mental health support to help her address her anxiety. If after discussion and offer of support, a vaginal birth is still not an acceptable option, offering a planned caesarean section is recommended (NICE, 2011).

baby might feel compelled to constantly check on the infant's wellbeing; for example, a fear of contamination by infection or a substance may lead to excessive cleaning rituals. Some sufferers of OCD have a compulsive need for symmetry or orderliness, which might be difficult to fulfil when having small children. Finally, and particularly frightening or repulsive for

Box 1.7 Practice learning point

- Obsessive compulsive disorder (OCD) in a mother without co-morbid impulse control problems or other significant co-morbidities, for example, substance misuse, personality disorder or psychosis, is unlikely to be a direct risk to the child.
- People with a family history of OCD might be more at risk of developing this condition (RCPsyc, 2018), as well as those who are meticulous, anxious or have a very strong sense of responsibility.
- Some people have OCD co-morbid with other anxiety disorders, depression or an eating disorder.

Table 1.2: Other types of conditions that may relate to obsessive compulsive disorder

Hoarding disorder is when the sufferer chaotically accumulates a number of items, usually of little monetary value, and is unable to get rid of those which are no longer needed and might hold a strong opinion about why the items are necessary. This can lead to clutter and, in extreme circumstances, too little space left in the house. This can pose a health risk and might be a reason for safeguarding concerns. Hoarding can be associated with obsessive compulsive disorder (OCD), severe depression or schizophrenia (WHO, 2020).

Body dysmorphia is a condition related to OCD. The person affected is preoccupied with one or more flaws in his or her appearance that might be unnoticeable to others. It occurs mainly in adolescents or young adults. Treatment is similar to that of OCD.

From World Health Organization (WHO). (2020). *ICD-11 Mental health.* https://www.who.int/health-topics/mental-health#tab=tab_1.

the mother to experience, are intrusive thoughts of a sexual nature when looking after her baby (RCPsyc, 2018).

Posttraumatic stress disorder

Posttraumatic stress disorder (PTSD) is a condition that develops in some individuals following exposure to an extremely threatening or horrific event(s) such as a threat to life, sexual abuse or trafficking. Women can experience PTSD following birth, particularly if the labour has been difficult and resulted in an emergency caesarian section or difficult vaginal birth. It is more likely to occur in women with pre-existing anxiety and depression.

Women admitted to high-dependency or intensive care units and those suffering obstetric loss are at increased risk of developing PTSD. Other risk factors include women previously abused, those with unwell infants in neonatal units, stillbirth and those with serious medical conditions. This does not include women with pre-existing PTSD, for example, who have experienced diverse traumatic experiences. PTSD is considered a remitting condition, but it can have a chronic course, too.

While the formal diagnosis of PTSD requires an objective threat to life situation (according to the WHO or American classification), symptoms of PTSD might also develop after experiencing a *perceived* threat to one's own or the infant's health or life. This might be because of prolonged, very painful and/or assisted labour, or the experience of emergency caesarean section (Furuta et al., 2018). A negative experience of the care received during labour or postnatally and feelings of powerlessness or lack of control during labour can all contribute to the subsequent development of psychological problems postnatally (Reed, Sharman, & Inglis, 2017). Symptoms that manifest in this way post-birth are called *birth trauma* and, in some instances, might be incorrectly labeled as postnatal depression or anxiety. Birth trauma can negatively affect bonding between the mother and baby (Simpson & Catling, 2016).

Symptoms of PTSD can also develop in birth partners after witnessing a difficult labour and/or birth (Etheridge & Slade, 2017). Other significant life events, for example, particularly acrimonious relationship breakups, can cause PTSD symptoms, too.

Symptoms of posttraumatic stress disorder

- Re-experiencing the traumatic event in the form of vivid intrusive memories, flashbacks or nightmares.
- Avoidance of thoughts and memories of the event or events, or avoidance of activities, situations or people reminiscent of the event or events (in the case of birth trauma, the woman might start avoiding hospital appointments or avoid looking at pictures of babies).
- Persistent perceptions of heightened current threat (hypervigilance, startle reaction, insomnia).
- Low mood and feelings of guilt or blame.

Complex posttraumatic stress disorder (complex PTSD) may develop following exposure to prolonged or repetitive events from which escape is difficult or impossible (e.g. torture, slavery, genocide campaigns, prolonged domestic violence, repeated childhood sexual abuse or physical abuse).

Box 1.8 Practice learning point

> The midwife should support women with posttraumatic stress disorder (PTSD) by facilitating a detailed discussion of birth options and careful birth planning. It is important that women with PTSD feel a sense of control during labour and birth; therefore the midwife should advocate for the woman where required to ensure that this is achieved.

Box 1.9 Practice learning point

> Adjustment disorder around the time of childbirth is very common. One study from Ireland found that out of 45 women attending a perinatal mental health service, almost half (48.9%) received a diagnosis of adjustment disorder (Doherty, Crudden, Jabbar, Sheehan, & Casey, 2019).

The symptoms are that of PTSD, but additionally the person suffers from:

- severe and long-term problems in affect regulation;
- feelings of worthlessness, shame, guilt or failure related to the traumatic event and
- difficulties sustaining relationships and feeling close to others.

Adjustment disorder

Adjustment disorder is a common mental health problem. It is diagnosed when a person develops excessive worries and is preoccupied with a stressful event, situation or life change, as well as its meaning and consequences, and finds it difficult to adapt to the change and cope. The condition can follow stressful life events such as significant relationship problems, divorce, illness, financial issues, job loss, etc. The disorder usually resolves within about 6 months, and adaptation to the life change follows. Adjustment can also take longer to occur if the stressor continues to be present, for example, continuing unemployment.

Symptoms are usually similar to those occurring in milder anxiety disorders, and depression or anger can also be present.

Attention-deficit/hyperactivity disorder

Attention-deficit/hyperactivity disorder (ADHD) is a neurodevelopmental disorder emerging in childhood, but in 65% of those affected, some impairment persists into adulthood. It occurs in 4 out of 100 people and is four times more frequent in boys than in girls. While children will often have symptoms of inattention and hyperactivity-impulsivity, in adults, symptoms may be more frequently associated with inattention (attention-deficit disorder or ADD), and hyperactivity becomes significant restlessness.

ADHD is highly co-morbid with other mental health problems, particularly with anxiety and depression. Women with ADHD suffer from poor concentration and impulsivity and might have problems with parenting. Untreated or inadequately treated ADHD can result in risk-taking, which may potentially place the mother and child at risk, both antenatally and postnatally. There is also an association between ADHD and substance misuse, but some evidence suggests that adequate treatment of ADHD may reduce this and help prevent co-morbidities (Katzman, Bilkey, Chokka, Fallu, & Klassen, 2017). Impulsivity can increase the risk of unplanned pregnancy.

Eating disorders

Eating disorders (EDs) are diagnosed when behaviours associated with weight control are linked to self-esteem and self-worth. EDs usually develop in adolescence and young adulthood and are more common among women (RCPsyc, 2018). The prevalence of anorexia nervosa is an estimated 7 per 1000 in the United Kingdom, with more incidences in adolescent girls and young women (Sebastiani et al., 2020). Bulimia nervosa is more frequent and affects older age groups, with a prevalence of 0.5%–1% in women of reproductive age (Sebastiani et al., 2020). In pregnancy, up to 7.5% of women may suffer from an ED (Easter et al., 2013). Binge eating and EDs, which have a less typical picture, are called 'non-otherwise specified'. It is estimated that approximately 5% of women may suffer with binge eating and non-otherwise specified EDs. Therefore it could be suggested that the prevalence of EDs among pregnant women are relatively commonplace but perhaps under-detected.

EDs have multi-factorial causality, and sociocultural, biological and psychological factors all contribute to the onset of this condition, including personality traits. It is worth noting that the condition can change over time from one presentation to another. For example, it is not unusual for a person to experience periods of anorexia followed by bulimia or vice versa. It is also not unusual for individuals with EDs to have personality difficulties with obsessive (anankastic) and anxious features.

Anorexia nervosa is diagnosed when body weight, that is body mass index (BMI), is 17.5 or less and the sufferer employs one or more methods to induce weight loss or not to put on weight.

This might include:

- restricted eating and dieting–purging;
- excessive exercising and
- using appetite suppressants, laxatives and/or diuretics.

The person suffering with anorexia tends to have a distorted body image pursuing thinness, has a fear of putting on weight ('fear of fatness') and/or has a preoccupation with losing weight that becomes overvalued and can be a source of dread. The resulting undernutrition can cause secondary endocrine and metabolic changes, including amenorrhea. Purging (which might be present both in anorexia and bulimia) can cause electrolyte imbalances and other physical problems, such as muscular weakness, bradycardia, cardiac arrhythmias and epileptic seizures. Anorexia, therefore, can affect fertility; however, some women who wish to have a child are motivated to put on weight to be able to conceive.

In atypical anorexia, the BMI can be higher than 17.5 and fertility maintained, while the overall symptoms (as discussed above) remain the same.

Bulimia nervosa is diagnosed when there are repeated episodes of over-eating (binge eating), followed by compensatory methods and significant preoccupation with the control of body weight aimed at reaching a set weight (which is acceptable to the person but is usually below a healthy weight). The person employs various methods to reduce the effects of binge eating including purging, exercising, dieting and very restrictive eating or fasting.

If a person's weight is normal or excessive but there are typical features of binge eating followed by guilt and restricted eating and other methods to reduce weight, the diagnosis is atypical bulimia nervosa.

Binge eating is when the person suffers bouts of over-eating, frequently managing stress in this way, but does not diet excessively or have other symptoms as described above. Binge eating can cause obesity.

Psychological over-eating can follow traumatic or stressful life events and can lead to obesity. Obesity per se can also be a source of psychological problems.

Little is known about the onset of EDs during pregnancy, but it is worth taking into account that historical EDs might resurface due to weight changes; however the illness can also improve in pregnancy.

EDs and weight changes in pregnancy can have a negative impact on pregnancy course and birth outcomes (Dorsam et al., 2019). Depending on the subtype of ED, the consequences for pregnancy appear to be different. Complications that have been observed in women with anorexia

Box 1.10 Practice learning point

- In more generalised behavioural disorders, such as severe personality disorder, eating disorders (ED) might be a part of the wider clinical picture of dysfunctional coping strategies to regulate emotional states.
- EDs, particularly if not treated early, can have chronic course and are difficult to treat. They can follow a remitting-relapsing pattern. There is a risk of premature mortality.
- Some women with an eating disorder will also suffer with perinatal anxiety and depression, which can both have a negative impact on pregnancy outcomes.

due to being underweight pre-pregnancy and insufficient weight gain during pregnancy include hypothermia, hypotension, hypertension, miscarriages, caesarean section, premature birth and reduced intrauterine growth restriction (Dorsam et al., 2019; Eagles, Lee, Raja, Millar, & Bhattacharya, 2012; Koubaa, Hallstrom, Lindholm, & Hirschberg, 2005; Micali, Simonoff, & Treasure, 2007).

For women with bulimia, there appears to be an increased risk of hyperemesis, microcephaly and small for gestational age.

Food intake and nutrition is important during pregnancy, and nutrients and vitamin deficiencies may be associated with neural tube defects in babies. It has been observed that mothers with ED are two times more likely to consume more than 350 mg/day (2500/week) or 25 cups of coffee per week compared with healthy women (Dorsam et al., 2019). This high caffeine consumption could be due to their desire to suppress appetite.

While weight gain can be beneficial for women with anorexia nervosa, it might be excessive in women with bulimia nervosa and binge eating. However, pregnancy could also have positive effect on women with bulimia, with the relaxation of restrictive eating pattern and reduction of symptoms, although relapse after birth is possible. Together with an increased risk of anxiety and depression after birth, women may have problems bonding with their babies, in which case skin-to-skin and breastfeeding may be helpful.

Box 1.11 Practice learning point

- Some women with EDs also misuse alcohol or drugs such as stimulants, which are another well-known risk factor for fetal development.
- Bonding with the pregnancy can be negatively affected, and fetal movements can be met with fear or disgust.

Box 1.12 Practice learning point

Many women with ED will be willing to eat 'for the baby' and engage with advice and treatment because of the change in motivation. It is important to give information about the risks that active EDs can have on pregnancy outcomes in an individualised and sensitive manner. Women can be ashamed of their problems, as well as being very anxious when changing their eating patterns to accommodate pregnancy status. Some women might be terrified that they will harm the baby by their behaviour.

1. If a woman declines weighing it is important to sensitively negotiate with her rather than engage in confrontation, remembering that she is very likely terrified.

Box 1.13 Practice learning point

> Any woman with a low body mass index who is not putting on weight in pregnancy, who has unexplained electrolyte imbalance or hypoglycaemia or who is excessively worried about weight or diet should be sensitively asked about problems with eating. If problems are identified, referral for treatment to an eating disorder service is required. NICE (2017) recommends assessment and treatment at the earliest opportunity.

The National Institute of Clinical Excellence (NICE) (2017) recommends:

- monitoring the woman's condition carefully throughout pregnancy and the postnatal period,
- assessing the need for fetal growth scans,
- discussing the importance of healthy eating during pregnancy and the postnatal period in line with the guideline on maternal and child nutrition and
- advising on feeding the baby in line with the guideline on maternal and child nutrition and supporting the woman with her feeding choice.

NICE (2017) recommends ED services for people with anorexia who have declined or do not want treatment and who have severe or complex problems. ED services should provide support, including psychoeducation about the disorder and monitoring of weight, mental and physical health and any risk factors, with coordination between services and involvement of the person's family members or caregivers (as appropriate).

Personality disorder

Personality disorder (PD) usually emerges in late adolescence and early adulthood, when one's personality is considered fully formed (Bach & First, 2018). The prevalence of PD is estimated in Western countries at approximately 12% (Marshall, Jomeen, Huang, & Martin, 2020). However, global epidemiological data appear to be fraught with inconsistencies; therefore it is difficult to predict the worldwide incidence of this condition within the general population (Marshall et al., 2020).

PD is usually diagnosed when issues persist for 2 or more years. Problems include low self-worth, inaccurate or unstable self-view, difficulties developing and maintaining close relationships and difficulties in the ability to understand others' perspectives and manage conflict in relationships (Bach & First, 2018). Symptoms are usually apparent in social interactions with others rather than reported by the sufferer.

There is a spectrum of severity, and while some people have personality difficulty that affects some areas of their lives only and is thus a milder problem, those with severe PD find it hard to function adaptatively in any area, cannot be in satisfactory relationships and might be not employable (Bach & First, 2018).

Some personality tendencies might be adaptive in certain circumstances; for example, attention to detail is welcome in accountancy but can also be seen as perfectionism and may be unrealistic to sustain in everyday life (thus is not adaptive). Other tendencies are not adaptive; for example, when a mother expects her baby to wake up every night at the same time or develop according to the exact details of a textbook, and, consequently, when this does not happen, she becomes distressed. The core of PD, therefore, lies in *more rigid ways of being* in a variety of personal and social situations.

For a diagnosis to be made, the problem needs to be generalised. This means issues manifest in a variety of personal and social situations, are not confined to a specific relationship or role and are associated with significant distress and poor functioning in a few areas of a person's life (personal, school, work, community).

The problem is usually in one or more of the following domains (*traits*):

- *Negative affectivity* – negativism, low self-esteem, distrustfulness
- *Detachment* – preference for maintaining social and/or personal distance from others, aloofness
- *Dissociality* – disregard for the rights and feelings of others, lack of empathy
- *Disinhibition* – irresponsibility, impulsivity, recklessness
- *Anancastia* – perfectionism, stubbornness and inflexibility, risk avoidance
- *Borderline pattern* – pervasive pattern of instability of interpersonal relationships, self-image and affects and marked impulsivity

Box 1.14 Practice learning point

Childbearing women with avoidant, dependent and obsessive-compulsive personality disorders have an increased risk of major depression during the postpartum period.

It is not unusual for the person with personality disorder (PD) to come into contact with mental health services for the first time with 'anxiety and depression', as both are frequently co-morbidities, as well as substance misuse. People with PD have an increased risk of death because of homicide, suicide or accidents.

(WHO, 2020)

In mental health services, the most commonly diagnosed PD is emotionally unstable personality disorder (EUPD), otherwise known as borderline personality disorder (BPD).

BPD is a serious mental illness, with periodic or regular risk to the self and burdened with premature mortality. Severe PD is associated with disturbances in mother–infant interaction, child safeguarding concerns and loss of custody. The person with BPD has significant fear and makes a frantic effort to avoid real or imagined abandonment or rejection. The person might experience heightened emotional states, anger and desperation when feeling rejected by others (e.g. being furious with a friend who did not take a call). The person engages in very unstable, intense relationships which tend to be short-lived. There is a chronic feeling of emptiness, self-hatred, persistent unstable self-image or sense of self and tendency to indulge in risky behaviours, including substance misuse and sexual behaviours. In the moment of heightened stress, the person might self-harm impulsively (which has a variety of meanings, such as intention to calm down or self-punish but also to take one's own life). There might be a tendency towards intense anger or difficulty controlling anger. Some people with BPD can experience transient dissociative symptoms or psychotic-like features in situations of high affective arousal.

It is thought that BPD results from both genetic factors (twin studies have estimated the heritability of BPD and BPD traits to be 30%–40%) and very difficult experiences such as child abuse, including child sexual abuse and neglect. Prenatal exposure to maternal stress in pregnancy (including severe traumatic stress such as death or suicide of a close relative, maternal loss or rape during pregnancy), exposure to drugs and tobacco smoking and maternal medical conditions all increase the long-term risk of BPD (Brannigan et al., 2020; Schwarze et al., 2013) and other severe mental illnesses. In particular, severe maternal stress in pregnancy has been linked with an almost 10 times increase of the risk of BPD in offspring some 30 years later (Brannigan et al., 2020). Growing up in a household with significant mental health problems and substance misuse can be another factor.

Women with BPD and other PDs marked with impulsivity and lack of planning are at risk of unplanned pregnancy. Erratic engagement with mental health services is not unusual, and attendance to emergency departments might be the main way of accessing help for some (in crisis only). There has been considerable progress in effective treatments available for people with severe PDs in the last 20 years. However, the initial phase, which is constructively engaging the person with psychological treatment, can take some time.

A large recent Swedish study found that nulliparous women with PD had a higher risk of mortality than those with PD and a childbearing

Box 1.15 Practice learning point

Pregnancy and the period after birth is a window of opportunity, taking into account increased motivation and the number of routine clinical encounters with maternity services.

Box 1.16 Practice learning points

- Women with personality disorders (PDs) benefit from seeing the same practitioner(s).
- Containing stance can be very helpful, coupled with sensitive boundary setting when faced with unreasonable demands. While some patients with PD can be described as difficult, it is important not to be reactive. High levels of anxiety and insecurity are usually hidden behind hostility and anger.
- Women with borderline personality disorder (and other personality disorders) might have a history of significant abuse and neglect and resulting unresolved trauma; **trauma-informed care** is highly recommended.
- If they are not under the care of mental health services already, most people would benefit from the referral because there is increased risk of depression and postnatal anxiety.
- Monitoring for safeguarding problems is required for both the child and adult.
- If a woman receives services from a few organisations, collaborative multi-agency work and good communication is needed.

history, for both natural and unnatural deaths (Kouppis, Bjorkenstam, Gerdin, Ekselius, & Bjorkenstam, 2020). One of the main features of BPD is the pervasive feeling of emptiness. In this group, the feeling of meaningfulness in life has been found to play a buffering role against hopelessness and to be a protective and preventive factor for suicide, and childbearing contains substantial meaning components.

Women with BPD during pregnancy have been found to be at increased risk of gestational diabetes, premature rupture of the membranes, chorioamnionitis, venous thromboembolism, caesarean section and preterm birth (Pare-Miron, Czuzoj-Shulman, Oddy, Spence, & Abenhaim, 2016). They may experience distress when touched, anticipate birth as traumatic and frequently request early delivery. Co-morbidity with substance abuse is common.

Severe mental illness

Severe mental illness (SMI) includes schizophrenia, bipolar disorder and other psychoses, complex and severe depression, as well as severe OCD and other anxiety disorders.

People with SMI have psychological problems that may have a severe impact on their ability to engage in functional and occupational activities; therefore active illness can have negative effects on parenting skills and functioning as a mother. Individuals with SMI have higher rates of physical ill-health than the general population and higher rates of health-risk behaviours, including obesity and tobacco smoking (approximately twice as high as that of the general population), and are likely to have long-term physical conditions.

Childbirth is associated with a small risk of developing a serious mental illness, such as postpartum psychosis and severe depressive illness, as well as an increased risk of relapse, particularly of BAD and severe depression. In pregnant women with bipolar illness who discontinued their medication, the relapse rate was reported as high as 85% (Austin, Highet, & the Expert Working Group, 2017). Chronic, long-standing, serious mental illness such as schizophrenia can worsen or recur during pregnancy and the postpartum period. However, the majority of acute-onset serious perinatal disorders present as a psychiatric emergency in the days and weeks following childbirth.

NICE (2017) recommends being alert for possible symptoms of postpartum psychosis in the first 2 weeks after childbirth if a woman has any past or present SMI or there is a family history of severe perinatal mental illness in a first-degree relative. If a woman has sudden onset of symptoms suggesting postpartum psychosis, she should be referred to a mental health service for immediate assessment (within 4 hours of referral).

Between 28 and 32 weeks of pregnancy, women with SMI should have a written care plan, developed by professionals in mental health services

Box 1.17 Practice learning point

Detection NICE (2017)
At a woman's first contact with services in pregnancy and the postnatal period, ask about:
- any past or present severe mental illness (SMI),
- past or present treatment by a specialist mental health service including inpatient care and
- any severe perinatal mental illness in a first-degree relative (mother, sister or daughter).

Referral to a specialist perinatal mental health service for assessment and treatment should be made for all women who:
- have or are suspected to have SMI or
- have any history of SMI (during pregnancy or the postnatal period or at any other time).

The woman's general practitioner should be informed of any referral made to perinatal mental health services.

(including specialist perinatal mental health services) and agreed in collaboration with the woman, her partner, her family and/or her caregiver. The plan should cover pregnancy, childbirth and the postnatal period (including the potential impact of the illness on the baby). It should include the following information:

- Treatment goals
- How outcomes will be routinely monitored
- Increased contact with specialist PMI services
- The names and contact details of key professionals

The care plan should be recorded in all versions of the woman's notes (her own records and maternity, primary care and mental health notes) and a copy given to the woman and all involved professionals.

BAD ('manic depressive illness') is diagnosed when a person has suffered at least two episodes of significantly disturbed mood and activity, with at least one episode of mania or hypomania. Episodes can include affective psychosis.

Episodes of elated mood are shorter, and depressive episodes might last 6 or more months. BAD occurs in about 1 in 100 of the general population and usually develops in early adolescence or young adulthood.

For symptoms of depression, see the beginning of this chapter under the heading 'Depression'.

Symptoms of mania

- *Elated mood* – mood that is out of keeping with individual circumstances; almost uncontrollable excitement in its most severe form
- *Increased activity* – in severe form the person will speak very quickly and jump from one subject to another ('pressure of speech')
- *Reduced need for sleep and food intake*, combined with increased energy and reduced hunger, and increased sexual drive
- *Inflated self-esteem and grandiosity* – sometimes with irritability, anger or suspiciousness towards others (e.g. 'angry mania')
- *Perceptual disturbances* – colours perceived as more vivid and pleasurable
- *Mild form of mania* – hypomania, might be more difficult to detect as good mood and good energy might be seen as positive and thus not reported
- *Risk taking* – increased alcohol intake, drug use, reckless money spending or plans, behaviours inappropriate to the circumstances

Puerperal psychosis (PP) is a **psychiatric emergency**, and symptoms usually present in the first 2 weeks (approximately 95%) after birth. It can be a first episode of psychosis or a relapse of pre-existing mental illness (usually BAD).

Box 1.18 Practice learning point

> If a woman suffered puerperal psychosis or depression in previous pregnancies, there is a very high risk of re-occurrence in subsequent pregnancies (Florio et al., 2018).

Box 1.19 Practice learning point

> Be aware that psychotic illnesses are associated with an increased rate of stillbirths and neonatal deaths.

Symptoms present rapidly after birth, with mood fluctuation, confusion and marked cognitive impairment suggestive of delirium, bizarre behaviour, insomnia, visual and auditory hallucinations and unusual (i.e. tactile and olfactory) hallucinations.

Women with BAD are particularly vulnerable to developing psychotic and non-psychotic episodes in the postpartum period (Florio et al., 2018). Sleep deprivation and interference with circadian rhythms during late pregnancy, during labour and during frequent newborn feeding promote mood destabilisation (Bergink, Rasgon, & Wisner, 2016). Constant care for the newborn is a major stressor, particularly where psychosocial and physical support is lacking.

The psychosocial consequences of psychotic and mood episodes during childbearing include an increased risk for substance use, smoking and high-risk behaviours that increase exposure to sexually transmitted infections, violence, victimisation, poor nutrition, non-compliance with medical care and alienation from social support systems.

Women with BAD are more often smokers (Vermeulen et al., 2019), overweight (Reilly-Harrington, Feig, & Huffman, 2018) and alcohol or substance abusers (Etain et al., 2017). Therefore it is not easy to study the illness directly and its outcomes on infants due to increased confounding factors. However, BAD has been associated with an increased risk of caesarean birth, instrumental birth and induction as well as preterm birth (Rusner, Berg, & Begley, 2016).

Schizophrenia is characterised by distortions in thinking (delusions), language, perception (hallucinations), emotions (blunted or incongruent affect) and sense of self (e.g. the experience that one's feelings, impulses, thoughts, or behaviours are under the control of an external force). Cognition can be impaired. Psychotic experiences, for example, hallucinations (hearing voices) or/and delusions can occur episodically and can also be chronic.

It is estimated that at some point during their life, approximately 1 in 100 people will suffer an episode of schizophrenia (RCPsych, 2017).

Small studies have shown that mothers with schizophrenia are at disproportionately high risk for being single parents, in receipt of social care involvement and custody loss (Ranning, Laursen, Thorup, Hjorthj, & Nordentoft, 2016). There have been rare reports of pregnant women with schizophrenia having delusions around the foetus and denial of pregnancy, and in rare but tragic circumstances, suicide and infanticide.

There is a risk of relapse of psychosis in pregnancy and increased risk of psychosis postnatally; however, compared with BAD, the risk is more equally distributed in the year after birth. Apart from psychosis, which can carry a high risk to the self and/or others in any SMI, the concern regarding parenting in women with schizophrenia is the risk of unintentional neglect because of cognitive impairment and/or *negative symptoms*. These include blunted affect (it looks similar to flat affect in depression), poverty of speech, apathy, anhedonia, reduced social drive, loss of motivation and lack of social interest.

Women with schizophrenia are more likely to have adverse obstetric and neonatal outcomes, also because of lifestyle factors (e.g. smoking, alcohol and drug misuse, poor nutrition), medical morbidity (in particular diabetes mellitus, obesity and hypertension), social adversities (poverty, domestic violence) and poor antenatal care (Nguyen et al., 2013; Vigod et al., 2020).

The above risks mean that women with schizophrenia need increased support from services and their families. Good care planning involving family members can be a significant contributor towards 'good enough' parenting.

Conclusion

The scope of mental illness is vast and impossible to cover in one chapter. However, by providing this overview, it is hoped that readers will feel compelled to delve deeper into PMI to increase their knowledge and understanding around this important topic. The breadth of care midwives provide to women must extend further to include competence and confidence in PMI. Mental health has been pushed aside for too long. It is time to bring it to the forefront to close the gaps in service provision and to recognise that if we work hard to achieve this goal, we can help improve pregnancy and birth outcomes for *all* women.

POINTS FOR REFLECTION

- *You see a woman for her 28-week antenatal appointment and notice she has self-harm marks on her arms. She has never disclosed any mental health issues to you before. How would you approach this and what would be your main concerns?*
- *You see a woman who has a history of bipolar affective disorder. She is 36 weeks pregnant and has remained well during the pregnancy. She discloses that she has stopped taking her medication because she feels fine and she is worried about how the medication might affect her baby. How would you manage this situation and what would be your main concerns?*
- *You see a woman for her day 5 postnatal visit and you notice that she is talking a lot and appears to have lots of energy. What would be your concerns and how would you approach this situation?*

References

Austin, M. P., Highet, N., & the Expert Working Group. (2017). *Mental health care in the perinatal period: Australian clinical practice guideline*. Melbourne: Centre of Perinatal Excellence. https://www.cope.org.au/about/.

Bach, B., & First, M. B. (2018). Application of the ICD-11 classification of personality disorders. *BMC Psychiatry, 18*(351). https://bmcpsychiatry.biomed-central.com/articles/10.1186/s12888-018-1908-3.

Bergink, V., Rasgon, N., & Wisner, K. L. (2016). Postpartum psychosis: Madness, mania, and melancholia in motherhood. *American Journal of Psychiatry, 173*(12), 1179–1188. https://pubmed.ncbi.nlm.nih.gov/27609245/.

Biaggi, A., Conroy, S., Pawlby, S., & Pariante, C. M. (2016). Identifying the women at risk of antenatal anxiety and depression: A systematic review. *Journal of Affective Disorders, 191*, 62–77. https://www.ncbi.nlm.nih.gov/pmc/articles/PMC4879174/#bib90.

Brannigan, R., Tanskanen, A., Huttunen, M. O., Cannon, M., Leacy, F. P., & Clarke, M. C. (2020). The role of prenatal stress as a pathway to personality disorder: Longitudinal birth cohort study. *The British Journal of Psychiatry, 216*(2), 85–89.

Doherty, A. M., Crudden, G., Jabbar, F., Sheehan, J. D., & Casey, P. (2019). Suicidality in women with adjustment disorder and depressive episodes attending an Irish perinatal mental health service. *International Journal of Environmental Research and Public Health, 16*(20), 3970. https://www.ncbi.nlm.nih.gov/pmc/articles/PMC6843376/.

Dorsam, A. F., Preibl, H., Micali, N., Lorcher, S. B., Zipfel, S., & Giel, K. E. (2019). The impact of maternal eating disorders on dietary intake and eating patterns during pregnancy: A systematic review. *Nutrients, 11*(4), 840. https://www.ncbi.nlm.nih.gov/pmc/articles/PMC6521012/.

Dubber, S., Reck, C., Muller, M., & Gawlik, S. (2014). Postpartum bonding: The role of perinatal depression, anxiety and maternal-fetal bonding during pregnancy. *Archives of Women's Mental Health, 18*(2), 187–195. https://pubmed.ncbi.nlm.nih.gov/25088531/.

Eagles, J. M., Lee, A. J., Raja, E. A., Millar, H. R., & Bhattacharya, S. (2012). Pregnancy outcomes of women with and without a history of anorexia nervosa. *Psychological Medicine, 42*, 2651–2660. https://doi.org/10.1017/S0033291712000414.

Easter, A., Bye, A., Taborelli, E., Corfield, F., Schmidt, U., Treasure, J., & Micali, N. (2013). Recognising the symptoms: How common are eating disorders in pregnancy? *European Eating Disorders Review, 21*(4), 340–344. https://pubmed.ncbi.nlm.nih.gov/23495197/.

Etain, B., Lajnef, M., Henry, C., Aubin, V., Azorin, J. M., Bellivier, F., … Leboyer, M. (2017). Childhood trauma, dimensions of psychopathology and the clinical expression of bipolar disorders: A pathway analysis. *Journal of Psychiatric Research, 97*, 37–45. https://www.sciencedirect.com/science/article/abs/pii/S0022395617301620?via%3Dihub.

Etheridge, J., & Slade, P. (2017). "Nothing's actually happened to me.": The experiences of fathers who found childbirth traumatic. *BMC Pregnancy & Childbirth, 17*, 80. https://www.ncbi.nlm.nih.gov/pmc/articles/PMC5341171/.

Florio, A. D., Gordon-Smith, K., Firty, L., Kosorok, M. R., Fraser, C., Perry, A., … Jones, I. (2018). Stratification of the risk of bipolar disorder recurrences in pregnancy and postpartum. *British Journal of Psychiatry, 213*(3), 542–547. https://www.ncbi.nlm.nih.gov/pmc/articles/PMC6429257/.

Forray, A., Focseneanu, M., Pittman, B., McDougle, C. J., & Epperson, C. N. (2010). Onset and exacerbation of obsessive-compulsive disorder in pregnancy and the postpartum period. *Journal of Clinical Psychiatry, 71*(8), 1061–1068. https://pubmed.ncbi.nlm.nih.gov/20492843/.

Furuta, M., Horsch, A., Edmond, S. W. Ng, Bick, D., Spain, D., & Sin, J. (2018). Effectiveness of trauma-focused psychological therapies for treating post-traumatic stress disorder symptoms in women following childbirth: A systematic review and meta-analysis. *Frontiers in Psychiatry, 9*, 591. https://www.ncbi.nlm.nih.gov/pmc/articles/PMC6255986.

Heron, J., Craddock, N., & Jones, I. (2005). Postnatal euphoria: Are 'the highs' an indicator of bipolarity? *Review: Bipolar Disorder, 7*(2), 103–110. https://doi.org/10.1111/j.1399-5618.2005.00185.x. PMID: 15762850.

Heron, J., & Oyebode, F. (2011). Postpartum hypomania: Future perspective. *Neuropsychiatry, 1*(1), 55–60. https://www.jneuropsychiatry.org/peer-review/postpartum-hypomania-future-perspective-neuropsychiatry.pdf.

Hofberg, K., & Brockington, I. (2000). Tokophobia: An unreasoning dread of childbirth: A series of 26 cases. *The British Journal of Psychiatry, 176*, 83–85. https://doi.org/10.1192/bjp.176.1.83.

Katzman, M. A., Bilkey, T. S., Chokka, P. R., Fallu, A., & Klassen, L. J. (2017). Adult ADHD and comorbid disorders: Clinical implications of a dimensional approach. *BMC Psychiatry*, 17, 302. https://www.ncbi.nlm.nih.gov/pmc/articles/PMC5567978/.

Koubaa, S., Hallstrom, T., Lindholm, C., & Hirschberg, A. L. (2005). Pregnancy and neonatal outcomes in women with eating disorders. *Obstetrics and Gynecology*, 105, 255–260. https://doi.org/10.1097/01.AOG.0000148265.90984.c3.

Kouppis, E., Bjorkenstam, C., Gerdin, B., Ekselius, L., & Bjorkenstam, E. (2020). Childbearing and mortality among women with personality disorders: Nationwide registered based cohort study. *British Journal Psychiatry*, 6(e95), 1–6. https://uu.diva-portal.org/smash/get/diva2:1477375/FULLTEXT01.pdf.

Knight, M., & MBRRACE, U. K. (2019). *Saving lives, improving mothers' care. Lessons learned to inform maternity care from the UK and Ireland Confidential Enquiries into Maternal Deaths and Morbidity 2015-17*. Oxford: National Perinatal Epidemiology Unit, University of Oxford.

Leach, D. M., Marino, C., & Nikevic, A. V. (2019). An evaluation of the contribution of maladaptive attitudes specific to motherhood and metacognitions in perinatal depression. *Psychiatry Research*, 274, 159–166. https://pubmed.ncbi.nlm.nih.gov/30802687/.

Marcus, S. M., Flynn, H. A., Blow, F. C., & Barry, K. L. (2003). Depressive symptoms among pregnant women screened in obstetrics settings. *Journal of Women's Health (Larchmt)*, 12, 373–380.

Marshall, C. A., Jomeen, J., Huang, C., & Martin, C. R. (2020). The relationship between maternal personality disorder and early birth outcomes: A systematic review and meta-analysis. *International Journal of Environmental Research and Public Health*, 17(16), 5778. https://www.ncbi.nlm.nih.gov/pmc/articles/PMC7460127/.

Micali, N., Simonoff, E., & Treasure, J. (2007). Risk of major adverse perinatal outcomes in women with eating disorders. *British Journal of Psychiatry*, 190, 255–259. https://doi.org/10.1192/bjp.bp.106.020768.

Nguyen, T. N., Faulkner, D., Frayne, J. S., Allen, S., Hauck, Y. L., Rock, D., & Rampono, J. (2013). Obstetric and neonatal outcomes of pregnant women with severe mental illness at a specialist antenatal clinic. *The Medical Journal of Australia*, 199(3 Suppl.), S26–9.

National Institute of Clinical Excellence (NICE). (2014). *Antenatal and postnatal mental health: Clinical management and service guidance. Clinical guideline [CG192]*.

National Institute of Clinical Excellence (NICE). (2011). *Caesarean section. Clinical guideline [CG132]*. Published date: 23 November 2011. Last updated: 04 September 2019.

National Institute of Clinical Excellence (NICE). (2009). *Depression in adults with a chronic physical health problem: recognition and management.* [CG91]. https://www.nice.org.uk/guidance/cg91/resources/depression-in-adults-with-a-chronic-physical-health-problem-recognition-and-management-pdf-975744316357.

National Institute of Clinical Excellence (NICE). (2017). *Eating disorders: Recognition & treatment. Clinical guideline.* www.nice.org.uk/guidance/ng69.

O'Hara, M. W., & Wisner, L. (2014). Perinatal mental illness: Definition, description and aetiology. *Best Practice & Research: Clinical Obstetrics & Gynaecology,* 28(1), 3–12. https://doi.org/10.1016/j.bpobgyn.2013.09.002.

Pare-Miron, V., Czuzoj-Shulman, N., Oddy, L., Spence, A. R., & Abenhaim, H. A. (2016). Effect of borderline personality disorder on obstetrical and neonatal outcomes. *Reproductive Health,* 26(2), 190–195. https://www.sciencedirect.com/science/article/abs/pii/S1049386715001668.

Public Health England Guidance. (2019). *Mental health and wellbeing: JSNA toolkit - perinatal mental health.* https://www.gov.uk/government/publications/better-mental-health-jsna-toolkit/4-perinatal-mental-health.

Ranning, A., Laursen, T. M., Thorup, A., Hjorthj, C., & Nordentoft, M. (2016). Children of parents with serious mental illness: With whom do they grow up? A prospective, population-based study. *Journal of the American Academy of Child and Adolescent Psychiatry,* 55(11), 953–961. https://pubmed.ncbi.nlm.nih.gov/27806863/.

Reed, R., Sharman, R., & Inglis, C. (2017). Women's descriptions of childbirth trauma relating to care provider actions and interactions. *BMC Pregnancy & Childbirth,* 17, 21. https://www.ncbi.nlm.nih.gov/pmc/articles/PMC5223347/.

Reilly-Harrington, N. A., Feig, E. H., & Huffman, J. C. (2018). Bipolar disorder and obesity: Contributing factors, impact on clinical course, and the role of bariatric surgery. *Current Obesity Reports,* 7(4), 294–300. https://pubmed.ncbi.nlm.nih.gov/30368736/.

Royal College of Psychiatrists (RCPsyc). (2017). *Factsheet: Schizophrenia: Information for parents, carers and anyone who works with young people.* http://www.rcpsych.ac.uk/healthadvice/parentsandyouthinfo/parentscarers/schizophrenia.aspx.

Royal College of Psychiatrists (RCPsyc). (2018). *Mental health in pregnancy.* https://www.rcpsych.ac.uk/mental-health/treatments-and-wellbeing/mental-health-in-pregnancy.

Rusner, M., Berg, M., & Begley, C. (2016). Bipolar disorder in pregnancy and childbirth: A systematic review of outcomes. *BMC Pregnancy & Childbirth,* 16(1), 331. https://pubmed.ncbi.nlm.nih.gov/27793111/.

Schwarze, C. E., Mobascher, A., Pallasch, B., Hoppe, G., Kurz, M., Hellhammer, D. H., & Lieb, K. (2013). Prenatal adversity: A risk factor in borderline personality disorder? *Psychological Medicine,* 06, 1279–1291.

Sebastiani, G., Andreu-Fernandez, V., Barbero, A. H., Aldecoa-Bilbao, V., Miracle, X., Barrabes, E. M., … Garcia-Algar, O. (2020). Eating disorders during gestation: Implications for mother's health, fetal outcomes, and epigenetic changes. *Frontiers in Pediatrics, 8*, 587. https://www.ncbi.nlm.nih.gov/pmc/articles/PMC7527592/#B7.

Shakeel, N., Eberhard-Gran, M., Sletner, L., Slinning, K., Martinsen, E. W., Holme, I., & Jenum, A. K. (2015). A prospective cohort study of depression in pregnancy, prevalence and risk factors in a multi-ethnic population. *BMC Pregnancy & Childbirth, 15*, 5.

Sim, K., Lau, W. K., Sim, J., Sum, M. Y., & Baldessarini, R. J. (2016). Prevention of relapse and recurrence in adults with major depressive disorder: Systematic review and meta-analyses of controlled trials. *International Journal of Neuropsychopharmacology, 19*(2), pyv076. https://www.ncbi.nlm.nih.gov/pmc/articles/PMC4772815/.

Simpson, M., & Catling, C. (2016). Understanding psychological traumatic birth experiences: A literature review. *Women & Birth Journal of the Australian College of Midwives, 29*(3), 203–207. https://pubmed.ncbi.nlm.nih.gov/26563636/.

Vermeulen, J. M., Wootton, R. E., Treur, J. L., Sallis, H. M., Jones, H. J., Zammit, S., … Munafo, M. R. (2019). Smoking and the risk for bipolar disorder: Evidence from a bidirectional Mendelian randomisation study. *British Journal of Psychiatry, 218*(2), 88–94. https://pubmed.ncbi.nlm.nih.gov/31526406/.

Vigod, S. N., Fung, K., Amarty, A., Bartsch, E., Felemban, R., Saunders, N., … Brown, H. K. (2020). Maternal schizophrenia and adverse birth outcomes: What mediates the risk? *Social Psychiatry & Psychiatric Epidemiology, 55*(5), 561–570. https://pubmed.ncbi.nlm.nih.gov/31811316/.

World Health Organization (WHO). (2020). *ICD-11: Mental health*. https://www.who.int/health-topics/mental-health#tab=tab_1.

CHAPTER 2

Pharmacological interventions in perinatal mental health

Agnieszka Klimowicz and Michelle Anderson

Part 1: Risks and benefits of psychotropic medication

It is inevitable that most midwives will care for a woman taking medication for the treatment of mental illness at some point in their career. Therefore it is important that midwives have a basic knowledge of the types of pharmacological treatment available to ensure that women receive the best care possible throughout the pregnancy continuum. This chapter aims to give an overview of pharmacological treatments used in pregnancy and the risks and benefits to both mother and baby.

Introduction

Treatment of psychiatric disorders usually consists of a range of psychological, psychosocial and pharmacological interventions. For some, these interventions may be time-limited, for example 6 weeks of cognitive behavioural therapy (CBT) and/or a short course of antidepressants. However, others may require long-term medication for their psychiatric illness to prevent relapses and reoccurrences.

If a woman's mental state is stable while on medication(s) and she is considering having a child, it is advised that she receive pre-conception advice/counselling from a medical practitioner. This would usually be a general practitioner (GP), but in the case of women with significant mental health history and/or on a number of different types of medication, pre-conception advice should be provided by the community perinatal mental health teams.

It is important for women who are planning a pregnancy or for any woman who finds herself unexpectedly pregnant not to stop her medication suddenly. This is due to the potential for relapse and withdrawal effects. Some medications can have a teratogenic effect on the foetus (discussed later in this chapter); therefore it is important that the woman seeks prompt advice from either her perinatal mental health team or GP

Box 2.1 Practice learning point

> If a woman takes medication with known teratogenic risks, additional foetal screening might be required.

if she does become pregnant. Medication taken by the woman begins to enter the foetal circulation 13 days post conception (at the point when many women do not even know they are pregnant) (Göpfer, Webster, & Seeman, 2010) and has the potential to cause foetal abnormalities; therefore the woman may need to change her medication during pregnancy.

A planned pregnancy is likely to be healthier for the woman and her baby. Unplanned pregnancies represent a missed opportunity to optimise pre-pregnancy health in *all* women. Currently, 45% of pregnancies and one-third of births in England are unplanned or associated with feelings of ambivalence (PHE, 2018), which may be a contributing factor to the development of perinatal mental illness (PMI) in pregnancy and/or the postnatal period. The National Survey (2013) found that most unplanned pregnancies were in women aged 20–34 years (Wellings et al., 2013). Unplanned pregnancies may be higher in women with mental illness.

Public Health England (2018) points out a number of health behaviours associated with improved health in pregnancy which should be started in the pre-conception period:

+ being up to date with all vaccinations
+ ensuring sexual health checks and cervical screenings are up to date
+ taking vitamin D and folic acid supplements
+ eating a healthy, balanced diet and undertaking regular moderate-intensity physical activity
+ reducing alcohol consumption
+ giving up smoking
+ using contraception for family spacing
+ addressing the management of physical and mental health conditions, as well as social needs, allowing women to be aware of potential risks and make an informed decision about their pregnancies (PHE, 2018)

In pregnancy and the postnatal period, many mental health problems have a similar nature, course and potential for relapse compared with the non-pregnant population. However, there are also significant differences particularly in a range of more serious disorders. An example is an increased risk of relapse of bipolar affective disorder in the early weeks postnatally. Some alterations in mental health state and functioning (e.g. mood changes or food cravings due to pregnancy hormones) often represent normal pregnancy physiology; however, they may also be symptoms of a mental health problem (NICE, 2014).

Lifestyle factors have an important influence on mental health and pregnancy outcome and should be discussed during each antenatal and postnatal contact (see Chapter 7 for further details). Aside from the well-documented negative effects of poor diet, smoking and alcohol consumption, it is worth noting that moderate maternal caffeine consumption has been associated with low birth weight (Taylor, Barnes, & Young, 2018). Pre-pregnancy maternal obesity has been observed to increase the risk of neural tube defects (Taylor et al., 2018). All of these factors should be considered in order to gain a full picture of a woman's lifestyle habits and how they, along with medication for mental illness, may have an impact on the pregnancy and the infant.

The threshold for pharmacological interventions in pregnancy is higher as there is a changing risk–benefit ratio for psychotropic medication at this time. The woman should have a detailed discussion about her medication options with either her GP or a mental health professional to enable her to make an informed decision on reducing and/or stopping any current medication (NICE, 2014).

NICE (2014) recommends the following to be included in discussions with the woman

- the uncertainty about the benefits, risks and harms of treatments for mental health problems in pregnancy and the postnatal period
- the likely benefits of each treatment, taking into account the severity of the mental health problem
- the woman's response to any previous treatment
- the background risk of harm to the woman and the foetus or baby associated with the mental health problem and the risk to mental health and parenting associated with no treatment
- the possibility of the sudden onset of symptoms of mental health problems in pregnancy and the postnatal period, particularly in the first few weeks after childbirth (e.g. in bipolar disorder)
- the risks or harms to the woman and the foetus or baby associated with each treatment option
- the need for prompt treatment because of the potential effect of an untreated mental health problem on the foetus or baby
- the risk or harms to the woman and the foetus or baby associated with stopping or changing a treatment.

When a woman is first offered medication in pregnancy for her mental health, NICE (2014) recommends:

- choosing a drug with the lowest risk profile for the woman, foetus and baby, taking into account the woman's previous response to medication
- using the lowest effective dose (this is particularly important when the risks of adverse effects to the woman, foetus and baby may be dose-related)
- noting that sub-therapeutic doses may also expose the foetus to risks and not treat the mental health problem effectively
- using a single drug, if possible, rather than two or more drugs, taking into account that dosages may need to be adjusted in pregnancy.

Medication during breastfeeding

Treatment of PMI is particularly important after birth due to high risk of relapse and recurrence of mental health symptoms. Some new mothers might be anxious about whether the medication they are taking can transfer to the newborn via breast milk. It is beneficial to offer reassurance to the mother that most medications have only very small quantities present in breast milk and are unlikely to cause problems in the infant. Therefore breastfeeding is usually encouraged with very few exceptions. It is important that the woman be advised to continue taking her medication while breastfeeding.

A widely used measure for the estimation of risk of exposure to the baby from maternal psychotropic medication in breast milk is called relative infant dose (RID). RID estimates infant drug exposure via breast milk. When calculating RID, the milk concentration is used to estimate the amount of drug ingested by the infant (Elgnainy, 2018). Although midwives are not expected to calculate RID, it is useful to be aware of the method used to estimate exposure risk to the infant. If unsure, always discuss with a member of the paediatric team. This can be discussed with the paediatric team.

Estimated daily infant dose via breast milk (mg/kg/day) = drug concentration in breast milk (mg/mL) x volume breast milk ingested (mL/kg/day).

Box 2.2 Practice learning point

- If a woman decides to stop medication and she has a history of significant mental illness, there is a need for increased level of monitoring and support.
- Perinatal suicides are notable for being associated with a lack of active treatment, specifically treatment with psychotropic medications (Taylor et al., 2018).

When the actual volume for milk ingested by the infant is not known, 150 mL/kg/day should be used in the calculation (based on an exclusively breastfed infant) (Elgnainy, 2018).

Note: Dosing units (mcg, unit, gram, etc.) can be changed as appropriate.

If the RID is less than 10%, it is usually considered safe in breastfeeding (Elgnainy, 2018).

It is important to note that RID is an estimate, and it can vary between studies for the same medication. If there are any concerns, infants should be monitored for side effects and the paediatric team should be involved.

If the medication is associated with a risk of sedation, women should be advised that it might interfere with parenting and feeding at night. Women should also be advised not to breastfeed in bed when taking sedative medication to prevent the risk of falling asleep while feeding (Taylor et al., 2018).

Medication used to treat mental illness in pregnant women and during breastfeeding is unlicensed. This is predominantly because conducting robust research, such as randomised control trials to investigate safety, tolerability and efficacy, has ethical limitations in the pregnant population. However, there are a number of systematic reviews and prospective cohort studies offering data on outcomes from women taking psychotropic medication during pregnancy (Nyguen et al., 2013; Rusner, Berg, & Begley, 2016; Wisner et al., 2019). It is best to interpret this data with caution, however, because lifestyle and other confounding factors are not controlled for, which can result in bias for selective reporting of adverse outcomes.

PRACTICE LEARNING POINT

- If you encounter a woman who discloses she is taking psychotropic medication, at the booking appointment for example, and she has not discussed it with her doctor or received pre-conception advice, don't panic.
- The midwife should refer to a specialist team or GP, as appropriate. It is important to know your local perinatal mental health pathways, including referral criteria to your local community perinatal mental health team, and advice line numbers (if available).
- In the case of newly emerging symptoms, it is important for the midwife to screen for and explore those symptoms and refer as appropriate.
- Reassurance should be given to the woman if she is concerned.

- Avoid, whenever possible, negative language and absolute terms (e.g. 'harmful', 'safe', 'never' or 'always').
- Do not forget that for women with common mental health problems, a GP referral is appropriate. Local primary care improving access to psychological therapies (IAPT) services provide CBT and counselling for perinatal mental health issues.
- Secondary mental health services and specialist perinatal mental health services are required for more significant mental health concerns, including for those women who are currently well but have a significant psychiatric history (e.g. severe depression with a history of risk to self and/or others or severe impact on everyday functioning, bipolar affective disorder, schizophrenia, schizoaffective disorder, severe and/or chronic obsessive compulsive disorder (OCD), severe anxiety disorder including severe panic disorder).

Part 2: An overview of medications used for the treatment of mental health conditions

Antidepressants

Antidepressants are frequently defined as 'a group of medications used to treat depression'. This is a rather unusual definition given that antidepressants are also used for many other mental health conditions, including anxiety disorders, posttraumatic stress disorder (PTSD) and OCD. They are also used alongside other medications in severe mental illness, such as bipolar affective disorders or schizophrenia. They can also be used for physical health problems; for example, amitriptyline is sometimes used for the treatment of chronic pain.

Depression is the most common mental health condition at any time, including during pregnancy and after birth, and antidepressants are the most frequently used psychotropic medications. For this reason, more is known about antidepressants and their effects in pregnancy and on the neonate, especially selective serotonin reuptake inhibitors (SSRIs). The use of antidepressants in pregnancy is common in the United States (Taylor et al., 2018) and the rate is increasing. In the UK, a retrospective cohort study found that antidepressant prescribing in pregnancy increased nearly 4-fold from 1992 to 2006. However, during pregnancy most women did not receive further antidepressant prescriptions beyond 6 weeks' gestation (Petersen et al., 2011). This could be explained by concerns about potential adverse effects of the medication in pregnancy, even though these concerns need to be balanced against the potential harm of inadequate treatment of depression during pregnancy and the postnatal period (Petersen et al., 2011). For women who do discontinue antidepressants, the relapse rate is high, with one study reporting relapses in 68% of women who were previously well on antidepressants versus 26% of women who continued antidepressants in pregnancy (Cohen et al., 2006).

Although it is not fully understood how antidepressants work, it is known that they increase levels of certain neurotransmitters which are linked to mood and emotion in the brain – specifically serotonin and noradrenaline. The benefits of antidepressants on mental state are not usually apparent until after a few weeks of commencing treatment, and this delayed onset of action can result in an initial deterioration of mood. Additionally, all antidepressants may increase anxiety and agitation at the beginning of treatment, so close monitoring (weekly), particularly in younger people (under the age of 25), is recommended. This particular feature of antidepressant medication is important, as anxiety is a frequent symptom in perinatal depression. Therefore, on some occasions, antidepressants are combined with another type of medication on a temporary basis (such as benzodiazepine if the patient is post birth) to help alleviate anxiety and insomnia.

Some studies have reported that antidepressants can be associated with an increased risk of spontaneous abortion, pre-term delivery, low birth weight, respiratory distress and low APGAR scores in neonates (Adhikari, Patten, Lee, & Metcalfe, 2019; Cantarutti, Merlino, Monzani, Giaquinto, & Cottao, 2016; Eke, Saccone, & Berghella, 2016). However, most studies did not control for maternal depression and lifestyle factors. Maternal depression on its own has been associated with pre-term birth and babies who are small for gestational age (Liu, Cnattingius, Bergstrom, Ostberg, & Hjern, 2016). Antidepressants do not appear to increase the risk of stillbirth or neonatal mortality. While it appears that most antidepressants are not major teratogens, there are conflicting data about risk of cardiac malformations. There are also studies associating antidepressant use with positive outcomes, such as lower rates of caesarean section in women taking antidepressants compared with women with psychiatric illness who are not taking antidepressants (Taylor et al., 2018).

Antidepressant withdrawal syndrome (discontinuation syndrome)

Antidepressant withdrawal syndrome is seen in adults and can occur upon abrupt stopping or significant reduction of the dose of antidepressant, particularly if the medication was taken on a long-term basis. Symptoms are usually mild and may develop after treatment with any type of antidepressant (and other psychotropic medications). Symptoms usually become apparent within 2 to 4 days after drug cessation and last approximately 1 to 2 weeks (and occasionally may persist up to 1 year). If the same or a similar drug is started, the symptoms will resolve within 1 to 3 days (Gabriel & Sharma, 2017).

Antidepressant withdrawal syndrome may result in medical or psychiatric misdiagnosis, as the syndrome can produce flu-like symptoms (lethargy, fatigue, headache, achiness, sweating). Other symptoms are insomnia (with vivid dreams or nightmares), nausea dizziness, vertigo, light-headedness, sensory disturbances (burning, tingling, electric-like or shock-like sensations) and hyperarousal (anxiety, irritability, agitation, aggression, mania, jerkiness). Early pregnancy can be a time of anxiety which can cause a woman to stop taking her antidepressants without consultation with the prescriber. Therefore it is important that women receive information and advice about continuing to take medication and the potential consequences of failure to do so. Women should be advised that discontinuation syndrome is not a sign of addiction. Because discontinuation syndrome can also look like a relapse of psychiatric disorder, it can be erroneously interpreted this way by the person experiencing it. The best way to manage significant withdrawal syndrome is to increase the dose or restart the antidepressant at the dose which does not produce symptoms, and if the antidepressant is to be withdrawn, it should be slowly tapered for 6 to 8 weeks (but on occasion much longer time is required).

Poor neonatal adaptation syndrome

Poor neonatal adaptation syndrome (PNAS) occurs in an estimated 25%–30% of neonates after exposure to antidepressants in the third trimester (Forsberg, Navér, Gustafsson, & Wide, 2014; Pan-London Perinatal Mental Health, 2017). The aetiology remains unclear, but it appears similar to adult withdrawal syndrome. No treatment intervention is usually required. Symptoms include poor feeding, poor sucking, irritability, vomiting, diarrhoea, agitation, tremors, jitteriness, hyperreflexia, decreased tone, hypothermia, temperature instability, hypoglycaemia and increased respiratory rate. Symptoms usually occur between 8 and 48 hours following birth and resolve within 2–3 days. PNAS is usually a mild and transient condition, however a very small proportion of infants might suffer severe PNAS (Forsberg et al., 2014). If the baby is at home and symptoms are detected by the midwife, the infant should be admitted to the hospital for examination. The baby must be monitored for central nervous system, motor, respiratory and gastrointestinal symptoms (Pan-London Perinatal Mental Health, 2017).

Table 2.1: **Types of antidepressants**

Type of commonly used antidepressant (AD)	Pharmacological action and risk profile in pregnancy	Risk to foetus	Compatible with breastfeeding
Selective serotonin reuptake inhibitors (SSRIs). Includes citalopram, escitalopram, fluoxetine, sertraline, paroxetine, fluvoxamine	Side effects are somewhat different for each one. They may cause agitation or anxiety, indigestion, headaches, dizziness, dry mouth, sexual dysfunction, increased weight gain, etc. Sertraline is considered the preferred choice of antidepressant in pregnancy, especially in women who have not taken an AD previously (Taylor et al., 2018). All SSRIs increase the risk of bleeding. SSRIs can be taken during pregnancy and any risks should be discussed with the patient.	PNAS SSRI are not considered teratogenic but there have been some studies indicating a slightly increased risk of heart defects. Persistent Pulmonary Hypertension of the Newborn (PPHN).	Yes, thought to be low levels present in breast milk. Therefore, advice is to breastfeed unless other contradictions present (PAN-London, 2017).
Serotonin-noradrenaline reuptake inhibitors (SNRIs). Venlafaxine, duloxetine	Usually prescribed as a second choice or when the treatment of anxiety in depression is particularly important. Venlafaxine is associated with more significant withdrawal syndrome when stopped suddenly in adults.	PNAS	Yes; thought to be low levels present in breast milk. Therefore, advice is to breastfeed unless other contraindications present (PAN London, 2016).

(Continued)

Table 2.1: **Types of antidepressants—cont'd**

Type of commonly used antidepressant (AD)	Pharmacological action and risk profile in pregnancy	Risk to foetus	Compatible with breastfeeding
Mirtazapine. Tetracyclic antidepressant	Second-choice antidepressant. Fewer data available in pregnancy compared with SSRIs. It has a calming effect in low doses (7.5 mg or 15 mg), and it is sometimes used for anxiety or for insomnia. It becomes effective for depression at a dose of 30 mg daily.	PNAS	Yes; thought to be low levels present in breast milk. Advice is to breastfeed unless other contraindications present.
Tricyclic antidepressants (TCAs). Amitriptyline, imipramine, nortriptyline, clomipramine, doxepin, dosulepin, lofepramine	Produce more side effects than other antidepressants and can be cardiotoxic and fatal in overdose. Less frequently used at present.	PNAS	Yes; thought to be low levels present in breast milk therefore, advice is to breastfeed unless other contradictions present. Pan London, 2016

Omega-3 fatty acids

Omega-3 fatty acids are increasingly used to support mood stability in a range of psychiatric conditions. They are naturally occurring in food and can be used as a supplement in much higher doses (fish or krill oil, flaxseed oil). Adequate intake in pregnancy and during breastfeeding is encouraged. The use as a treatment for mental health requires much higher doses (minimum 1 g/day), and a recent meta-analysis of randomised controlled trials (RCTs) detected moderately positive effects on symptoms of mild to moderate perinatal depression (Zhang et al., 2020). Breastfeeding data are conflicting regarding the positive effects on infant development, with some studies reporting negative effects (Lactmed, 2020). As omega-3 fatty acids are classified as supplements, there is also a concern about contamination (heavy metals, bacteria and fungi) (Zhang et al., 2020).

Table 2.2: Brain stimulation non-pharmacological methods for treatment of depression

Type of treatment	Risk to pregnancy
Electroconvulsive therapy (ECT). Last resort treatment – rarely used. ECT is by far the most effective psychiatric treatment for potentially life-threatening mental states, and it is supported by NICE for such use (catatonia, prolonged and severe mania).	Risk associated with general anaesthesia (Taylor et al., 2018), and ECT can cause transient or long-term memory problems, which limit its use.
Repetitive transcranial magnetic stimulation (rTMS). Until recently, rTMS was used in academic centres and for research purposes mainly. It is an evidence-based treatment currently supported by NICE for treatment-resistant depression (but not in pregnancy). Availability in the NHS is very limited. Its effectiveness is comparable to that of ECT, and since the effects of rTMS are in the brain, the treatment does not appear to have peripheral side effects which frequently occur when chemical antidepressants are used (Stahl, 2013).	As rTMS safety seems to be good in comparison to antidepressants (there is however very small risk of epileptic fit), theoretically it could be a good fit for pregnancy and breastfeeding. However, literature is very scant with one case study and one small RCT in pregnancy (Kim et al., 2019; Tan et al., 2008).

Mood stabilizers

Mood stabilizers are a difficult to define group, for which lithium seems to be best known. They are used to treat mood disordered states – for example, to treat depression when it is important to reduce or eliminate the risk of switching to mania or for the treatment of mania in order to 'stabilize' mood.

Women who take antiepileptics (which are a group of medications also used as mood stabilizers, for example lamotrigine) should take folic acid 5 mg in the first trimester.

Table 2.3: **Mood stabilizers**

Type of mood stabilizer	Side effect profile	Pharmacological action and risk profile in pregnancy	Risk to foetus	Breastfeeding compatibility
Lithium	Requires regular monitoring, as its level in blood is associated with its effectiveness. High levels may also lead to toxicity which can occur due to dehydration caused by hyperemesis gravidarum, diarrhoea during infection or after excessive sweating. Side effects range from tremors, gastrointestinal tract symptoms, weight gain and hair loss to long-term adverse effects such as hypothyroidism or effect on kidney function. Lithium appears to be used less frequently now (Poels Bijma, Galbally, & Bergink, 2018).	Particularly effective in the treatment of manic episodes and in the maintenance of recurrence, particularly in prevention of mania. It is somewhat less effective in the prevention of depressive episodes. Lithium can be used in combination with an antidepressant to improve the clinical response in unipolar depression. NICE (2014) recommends considering stopping lithium in pregnancy. If lithium is continued in pregnancy, further NICE guidance is available on its management in pregnancy. Its levels change significantly in pregnancy and require monitoring.	Risk of cardiac malformations, including a rare condition: Ebstein anomaly. Recent studies indicate that while lithium appears to increase the risk of major malformations, it does not appear to significantly increase the risk of major cardiac malformations (Munk-Olsen et al., 2018). Neonatal goitre, hypotonia, lethargy and cardiac arrhythmia can occur (Taylor et al., 2018). Maximum risk to the foetus is between 2 and 6 weeks after conception.	In the first trimester, woman who take lithium or restart lithium after birth are advised not to breastfeed due to relatively high exposure risk of lithium via breast milk and the risk of toxicity (PAN London, 2016).

Lamotrigine	Lamotrigine is usually well tolerated. The main concern is regarding the risk of rashes and a very small risk of life-threatening Stevens-Johnson syndrome.	Antiepileptic medication, considered to have relatively good reproductive safety profile. Used for treatment of bipolar depression.	Appears not to increase the risk of major malformations in the foetus.	Infants are exposed to lamotrigine via breast milk and they can have relatively high serum levels. However, this is not a contraindication to breastfeeding. Mixed feeding can be also considered.
	Lamotrigine is therefore gradually introduced and increased slowly for a number of weeks.			Infants should be monitored for side effects such as apnoea, rash, drowsiness or poor sucking.
	Metabolism of lamotrigine changes in pregnancy. Therefore maternal serum levels should be monitored and doses titrated as required.			Checking infant serum levels is advised. Breastfeeding should be discontinued if the infant develops a rash.

(Continued)

Table 2.3: Mood stabilizers—cont'd

Valproates are currently prohibited and must not be prescribed to women of childbearing age (unless the conditions of a pregnancy prevention programme are met). If valproate is taken during pregnancy, up to four in 10 babies are at risk of developmental disorders and approximately one in 10 are at risk of birth defects (Medicines & Healthcare Products Regulatory Agency (MHRA), 2018).

Carbamazepine should not be prescribed for women who are planning pregnancy or are pregnant due to the increased risk of major malformations (neural tube defects including spina bifida, cleft palate and other problems). Absolute risk estimates range from 3% to 10%. The risk appears to be dose-related, with higher risk if a mother takes 1000 mg daily or more (UKTIS, 2020). If a woman is advised to stop carbamazepine, it should be done gradually over a period of a few weeks.

Antipsychotics

Antipsychotics are a group of medications used for the treatment of psychotic conditions, such as schizophrenia. Newer antipsychotics, also called atypical antipsychotics, have mood stabilizing properties and are therefore also effective in the treatment for bipolar affective disorder. Lower doses of atypical antipsychotics can be added to antidepressants in treatment-resistant depression or are sometimes used to reduce heightened arousal, for example in emotionally unstable personality disorder or in the treatment of resistant anxiety disorders.

Benzodiazepines and Z-drugs

Benzodiazepines are commonly used for the temporary treatment of anxiety, some can be used for insomnia and Z-drugs are used for the short-term treatment of insomnia.

Anxiety is a common issue in pregnancy and after birth. If it is an isolated problem, psychological therapy and changes to lifestyle should be considered before pharmacological methods. However, if the symptoms affect day-to-day life and are sustained, anxiolytic (anti-anxiety) medication can be prescribed temporarily.

Please note: Promethazine, and not benzodiazepines or Z-drugs, is recommended by NICE for the treatment of significant anxiety and insomnia in pregnancy.

Attention-deficit/hyperactivity disorder (ADHD) is a common condition that might require treatment in adulthood (Poulton, Armstrong, & Nanan, 2018). As the awareness of ADHD is slowly growing, more women are taking stimulants (usually initiated by ADHD specialists) than ever before. An Australian population-based cohort study concluded that compared with no treatment, ADHD stimulant treatment at any time was associated with small increases in the risk of some adverse pregnancy outcomes (Poulton et al., 2018). Treatment before pregnancy, or before and during pregnancy, was associated with additional adverse outcomes, even after a treatment-free period of several years. However, none of these associations can be confidently attributed to stimulant treatment and further research is needed in this area (Poulton et al., 2018).

Table 2.4: Antipsychotic medications

Type of antipsychotic	Side effect profile	Pharmacological action and risk profile in pregnancy	Risk to foetus	Breastfeeding compatibility
Conventional (older) antipsychotics (APs). Includes haloperidol, chlorpromazine, flupentixol, trifluoperazine, zuclopenthixol.	Prone to produce extrapyramidal side effects (EPSEs), for example tremor, dystonia, slurred speech, akathisia and parkinsonism (e.g. bradyphrenia).	Typically used in the treatment of schizophrenia.	Do not seem to increase the risk of major malformations. Occasional reports of EPSEs in neonates Neonatal Pain, Agitation and Sedation (NPAS)	Yes, generally low levels in breast milk but limited data. Advice is to breastfeed unless other contraindications present.
Atypical antipsychotics (newer). Includes quetiapine, olanzapine, clozapine, amisulpride, ziprasidone, aripiprazole, lurasidone, risperidone	Associated with sedation and risk of metabolic syndrome (weight gain, increased blood pressure, dyslipidaemia, increased glucose level and diabetes).	Used for schizophrenia and bipolar affective disorder. If antipsychotic or mood stabilising medication is required in pregnancy, this group of medications is widely used. Women who are on antipsychotics in pregnancy should have a glucose tolerance test performed and be monitored for diabetes.	Quetiapine, aripiprazole or risperidone do not appear to be associated with an increased risk of major foetal malformations. Olanzapine has been associated with adverse pregnancy outcomes, including neonatal death due to cardiovascular defect and abortion (three therapeutic, one spontaneous) (Creeley & Denton, 2019). PNAS Amisulpiride – less used and fewer data. Very little to no information on ziprasidone, lurasidone or cariprazine.	Data is very limited, quetiapine, olanzapine and aripiprazole are present in very small to small amounts in breast milk. Risperidone – low levels but higher than the above antipsychotics. Probably compatible with breastfeeding. Very little to no information on ziprasidone, lurasidone or cariprazine. Clozapine – little published information and risk of haematological effects; possibly best to avoid.

Table 2.5: **Anxiolytic medication & Hypnotics (Z-drugs)**

Type of anxiolytic	Side effect profile	Pharmacological action and risk profile in pregnancy	Risk to foetus	Breastfeeding compatibility
Benzodiazepines. Longer-acting – diazepam nitrazepam flurazepam alprazolam chlordiazepoxide clobazam clonazepam Shorter-acting – lorazepam temazepam oxazepam	Addictive potential so should not be used on long-term basis. If a woman who takes them regularly becomes pregnant, abrupt stopping might be problematic.	If benzodiazepines are used in pregnancy or breastfeeding, short-acting benzodiazepines are preferable (NICE, 2014).	Conflicting data about teratogenic effects. Regular use in the third trimester is associated with a risk of neonatal withdrawal syndrome and 'floppy baby syndrome'.	Shorter-acting benzodiazepines are recommended for breastfeeding. There is a risk of accumulation of longer-acting benzodiazepines in infant serum (e.g. diazepam) **Z-drugs** Low levels of zolpidem & zaleplon in breastmilk, therefore breastfeeding is advised unless other contraindications present. Little data on zopiclone therefore best to use alternative during pregnancy. (PAN London, 2017).
Z-drugs. Zopiclone, zolpidem, zaleplon	Should not be used on a regular basis in pregnancy.		May increase the risk of low birth weight and premature birth (Creeley & Denton, 2019).	

Table 2.6: Other medications

Type	Side effect profile	Pharmacological action and risk profile in pregnancy	Risk to foetus	Breastfeeding compatibility
Pregabalin	Should not be withdrawn abruptly. Headaches, feeling sleepy, dizziness, mood changes, weight gain, etc.	Anticonvulsant which is also used and licensed for the treatment of neuropathic pain and general anxiety disorder. Controlled drug in the UK. Limited information on effects in pregnancy.	Foetal toxicity was reported in animal studies. Risk of PNAS, and it is advisable for birth to take place in a unit with adequate neonatal facilities (UKTIS, 2020)	Presence in breast milk probably low but limited data.
Medications for ADHD Methylphenidate (Concerta)	Can be abused.	Mild central nervous system stimulant used to treat attention-deficit/hyperactivity disorder (ADHD).	Limited data indicate that it is not teratogenic.	Present in very low amounts in breast milk, based on limited data.

Conclusion

This chapter has presented a basic overview of the medication used in the treatment of PMI. It is merely a guide to encourage further reading and also to enable midwives to recognise psychotropic medication should they encounter it in clinical practice. It is worth remembering that women who require medication for their mental health may be anxious about its effect it on pregnancy. Therefore it is important that midwives are able to recognise this type of medication and offer reassurance to the mother and her family, should it be required. Ensuring robust clinical care pathways are in place for perinatal mental health, and with collaborative training in this ever-growing arena, we can all work synergistically to provide the best perinatal mental health care possible for mothers and babies.

References

Adhikari, K., Patten, S. B., Lee, S., & Metcalfe, A. (2019). Risk of adverse perinatal outcomes among women with pharmacologically treated and untreated depression during pregnancy: A retrospective cohort study. *Paediatric & Perinatal Epidemiology, 33*(5), 323–331. https://doi.org/10.1111/ppe.12576.

Cantarutti, A., Merlino, L., Monzani, E., Giaquinto, C., & Cottao, G. (2016). Is the risk of preterm birth and low birth weight affected by the use of antidepressant agents during pregnancy? A population-based investigation. *PLoS One.* https://www.ncbi.nlm.nih.gov/pmc/articles/PMC5158190/#:~:text=Our%20large%20population%2Dbased%20study,9%20months%20before%20pregnancy%20until.

Cohen, L. S., Altshuler, L. L., Harlow, B. L., Nonacs, R., Newport, D. J., Viguera, A. C., ... Stowe, Z. L. (2006). Relapse of major depression during pregnancy in women who maintain or discontinue antidepressant treatment. *JAMA, 295,* 499–507. https://jamanetwork.com/journals/jama/fullarticle/202291.

Creeley, C. E., & Denton, L. (2019). Use of prescribed psychotropics during pregnancy: A systematic review of pregnancy, neonatal, and childhood outcomes. *Brain Sciences.* https://www.ncbi.nlm.nih.gov/pmc/articles/PMC6770670/.

Eke, A. C., Saccone, G., & Berghella, V. (2016). Selective serotonin reuptake inhibitor (SSRI) use during pregnancy and risk of preterm birth: A systematic review and meta-analysis. *BJOG: An International Journal of Obstetrics & Gynaecology.* https://pubmed.ncbi.nlm.nih.gov/27239775/.

Elgnainy, H. (2018). Relative infant dose (RID). *PEDIAMCU.* http://www.pediamcu.com/2018/01/relative-infant-dose.html.

Forsberg, F., Navér, L., Gustafsson, L. L., & Wide, K. (2014). Neonatal adaptation in infants prenatally exposed to antidepressants- clinical monitoring using neonatal abstinence score. *PLoS One.* https://doi.org/10.1371/journal.pone.0111327.

Gabriel, M., & Sharma, V. (2017). Antidepressant discontinuation syndrome. *CMAJ*, *189*(21), E747. https://doi.org/10.1503/cmaj.160991.

Göpfer, M., Webster, J., & Seeman, M. V. (2010). Seem & Seeman: Psychopharmacology and motherhood. In *Parental Psychiatric Disorder Distressed Parents and their Families* (2nd ed.). Cambridge: Cambridge University Press.

McAllister-Williams, H., Baldwin, D. S., Cantwell, R., Easter, A., Gilvarry, E., & Glover, V., (2017). *British association for psychopharmacology consensus guidance on the use of psychotropic medication preconception, in pregnancy and postpartum. Journal of Psychopharmacology*, *31*(5), 519–552. https://doi.org/10.1177/0269881117699361.

Kim, D. R., Wang, E., McGeehan, B., Snell, J., Ewing, G., Iannelli, C., … Epperson, C. N. (2019). Randomized controlled trial of transcranial magnetic stimulation in pregnant women with major depressive disorder. *Brain Stimulation*, *12*(1), 96–102. Jan–Feb.

Liu, C., Cnattingius, S., Bergstrom, M., Ostberg, V., & Hjern, A. (2016). Prenatal parental depression and preterm birth: A national cohort study. *BJOG: An International Journal of Obstetrics & Gynaecology*. https://obgyn.onlinelibrary.wiley.com/doi/full/10.1111/1471-0528.13891.

Medicines & Healthcare Products Regulatory Agency (MHRA). (2018). Valproate use by women and girls – Information about the risks of taking valproate medicines during pregnancy. *Guidance: Medicines and Healthcare Products Regulatory Agency*, Last updated 6 May 2020.

Munk-Olsen, M., Liu, X., Viktorin, A., Brown, H. K., Florio, A. D., D'Onofrio, B. M., … Bergink, V. (2018). Maternal and infant outcomes associated with lithium use in pregnancy: An international collaborative meta-analysis of six cohort studies. *The Lancet Psychiatry*, *5*(8), 644–652.

Nguyen, T. N., Faulkner, D., Frayne, J. S., Allen, S., Hauck, Y. L., Rock, D., Rampono, J. (2013). Obstetric and neonatal outcomes of pregnant women with severe mental illness at a specialist antenatal clinic. *The Medical Journal of Australia*. https://pubmed.ncbi.nlm.nih.gov/25369845/.

Pan-London Perinatal Mental Health. (2017). *Guidance for newborn assessment by the pan london perinatal mental health network and the london neonatal operational delivery network*. http://www.londonneonatalnetwork.org.uk/wpcontent/uploads/2016/10/FinalNeodoc-v3.pdf

Petersen, I., Gilbert, R. E., Stephen, M. D., Evans, J. W., Man, S. I., & Nazareth, I. (2011). Pregnancy as a major determinant for discontinuation of antidepressants: An analysis of data from the Health Improvement Network. *Journal of Clinical Psychiatry*, *72*(7), 979–985. https://doi.org/10.4088/JCP.10m06090blu.

Poels, E. M. P., Bijma, H. H., Galbally, M., & Bergink, V. (2018). Lithium during pregnancy and after delivery: A review. *International Journal of Bipolar Disorders*, *6*(26). https://doi.org/10.1186/s40345-018-0135-7.

Poulton, A. S., Armstrong, B., & Nanan, R. K. (2018). Perinatal outcomes of women diagnosed with attention-deficit/hyperactivity disorder: An Australian population-based cohort study. *CNS Drugs*, 32(4), 377–386. https://doi.org/10.1007/s40263-018-0505-9.

Public Health England Guidance. (2018). *Health matters: Reproductive health and pregnancy planning*. Published 26 June 2018.

Rusner, M., Berg, M., & Begley, C. (2016). Bipolar disorder in pregnancy and childbirth: A systematic review of outcomes. *BMC Pregnancy & Childbirth*. https://bmcpregnancychildbirth.biomedcentral.com/articles/10.1186/s12884-016-1127-1.

Stahl, S. M. (2013). *Stahl's essential psychopharmacology: Neuroscientific basis and practical application* (4th ed.). Cambridge: Cambridge University Press.

Tan, O., Tarhan, N., Coban, A., Baripoglu, S. K., Guducu, F., Izgi, H. B., … Bulut, H. (2008). Antidepressant effect of 58 sessions of rTMS in a pregnant woman with recurrent major depressive disorder: A case report. *Prim Care Companion Journal of Clinical Psychiatry*, 10(1), 69–71.

Taylor, D., Barnes, T., & Young, A. (2018). *The Maudsley prescribing guidelines in psychiatry* (13th ed.). Spain: Wiley Blackwell.

UK Teratology Information Service (UKTIS). (2020). Best use of medicines in pregnancy. http://www.uktis.org/index.html

Wellings, K., Jones, K. G., Mercer, C. H., Tanton, C., Clifton, S., Datta, J., … Johnson, A. M. (2013). The prevalence of unplanned pregnancy and associated factors in Britain: Findings from the third National Survey of Sexual Attitudes and Lifestyles (Natsal-3). *Lancet*, 382(9907), 1807–1816. https://doi.org/10.1016/S0140-6736(13)62071-1.

Wisner, K. L., Sit, D., O'Shea, K., Bogen, D. L., Clark, C. T., Pinheiro, E., … Ciolino, J. D. (2019). Bipolar disorder and psychotropic medication: Impact on pregnancy and neonatal outcomes. *Journal of Affective Disorders*. https://www.ncbi.nlm.nih.gov/pmc/articles/PMC6548542/.

Zhang, M. M., Zou, Y., Li, S. M., Wang, L., Sun, Y. H., Shi, L., … Li, S. X. (2020). The efficacy and safety of omega-3 fatty acids on depressive symptoms in perinatal women: A meta-analysis of randomized placebo-controlled trials. *Nature: Translational Psychiatry*, 10(193), 1–9.

Other resources and further information

Useful information about data relating to medication effects in pregnancy and the neonate can be found at https://www.uktis.org.

Highly recommended

British Association for Psychopharmacology consensus guidance on the use of psychotropic medication pre-conception, in pregnancy and postpartum, 2017. https://www.bap.org.uk/pdfs/BAP_Guidelines-Perinatal.pdf

Medications and pregnancy

UK Teratology Information Service (UKTIS), which according to its website is 'the sole dedicated UK provider of evidence-based information on foetal risk following pharmacological and other potentially toxic pregnancy exposures'.

Public-friendly website called BUMPS (best use of medicines in pregnancy) (https://www.medicinesinpregnancy.org/) has freely available, patient-friendly leaflets, which can be printed.

UKTIS also provides detailed scientific information for health care professionals via the website https://www.toxbase.org. Health professionals can register and have access to the information from their mobiles. Information on Toxbase and BUMPS is regularly updated.

CHAPTER 3

Psychological concerns in pregnancy

Judith Ellenbogen, Jane Anderson and Michelle Anderson

Introduction

Pregnancy, birth and the postnatal period is a very important time physically and psychologically for both mother and baby. How they interact during this period can have a lasting impact on their relationship. The physical and psychological care from the mother or significant caregivers is important in how the infant learns to relate to others over the course of his or her lifetime. The internalising of relationships, whether these are positive (loving, nurturing) or negative (neglectful, abusive), may have an impact on future relationships as the infant moves through childhood and into adulthood. The importance of this early attachment and relational behaviour to the mother/caregiver is shown in the work of Bowlby, Winnicott and Melanie Klein and others from the object relational school of psychoanalysis (Bowlby, 1969; Klein, 1940; Winnicott, 1973; Chapter 6 provides further details of the parent–infant relationship).

For many women, the transition to motherhood will raise thoughts and feelings about themselves, their identity, how they were parented and what sort of a mother they would like to be. Many women, with support of partners, family and friends, parenting groups and other resources, will find a way and place to discuss the issues around this transition, and most will feel supported well enough. However, for some women, pregnancy may trigger psychological difficulties that they were unaware of, or may exacerbate pre-existing mental health conditions.

The importance of providing psychological support and interventions from women's health counselling and perinatal mental health services is crucial for women experiencing a range of mental health issues (Perinatal Mental Health Services for London, 2017). In our experience, women are often more open and available to seek counselling during their pregnancy and feel less stigmatised for doing so, particularly if the counselling service is part of the multi-disciplinary team. The provision of psychological support, at such an important time in a woman's and baby's life, plays a pivotal role in preventing future psychological breakdown.

This chapter will discuss the work we undertake in the women's health counselling service. It serves as an introduction to psychological concerns during pregnancy. This is a very complex area, and further in-depth reading is recommended to explore women's experiences beyond their family backgrounds. Other factors to consider are the woman's position in the world in terms of socioeconomics, race, gender, sexuality, disability and religion and how these interplay with family dynamics. The first section of the chapter will portray the types of women we see, the reasons for referral and the

Box 3.1 Who we see in the service

Young women in their late teens to women in their 40s
Women from all socioeconomic backgrounds
Women from a wide range of ethnic groups and religions
Asylum seekers and refugees
Women who identify as heterosexual and LGBTQ+
Disabled women
Women who have a partner and single women

Box 3.2 Historical reasons for referral

Previous mental health problems (e.g. anxiety, depression, eating disorder, post traumatic stress disorder)
Previous loss of a baby through miscarriage, termination or stillbirth
Previous traumatic birth
Complications in previous pregnancy
History of sexual abuse, domestic violence and safeguarding issues
Discrimination based on race, gender, sexuality, disability or religion
History of postnatal depression
History of complex relationships and difficulties with attachment

Box 3.3 Concerns that may emerge during pregnancy

Phobias about childbirth, fears of invasive procedures and fears of physical changes in pregnancy
Fears of becoming a parent
Ambivalence about the pregnancy; fears of loss of professional identity, status and financial independence
Relationship changes
Experiences relating to discrimination based on race, gender, sexuality, disability or religion
Isolation, lack of family and friendship network
Antenatal depression and/or anxiety
Lack of material resources (e.g. inadequate housing, homelessness, lack of finances)
Religious and cultural issues and differences

underlying theoretical framework used in our counselling. The second section offers three case studies highlighting the kind of work we do and how it can be helpful. The next sections will discuss methods of evaluation and the place of the multi-disciplinary team, supervision and reflection.

Women are referred for a variety of reasons, some of which will pre-date the pregnancy, and others will be because of concerns that have emerged as a response to the pregnancy.

Theoretical models

Psychodynamic approach

Whilst there are a number of forms of therapy that could be effective in working with women during pregnancy, we use a psychodynamic approach as our basis, with particular reference to attachment and relational theory. This work draws on Freud, the object relations school of Melanie Klein and relational psychoanalysis (see Spurling, 2004, for a good introduction to this approach).

We also draw on cognitive behavioural therapy theory and techniques as this gives women clear strategies for managing symptoms (Greenberger & Padesky, 1995; Westbrook, Kennedy, & Kirk, 2007).

The fundamental premise of psychodynamic counselling is that responses to relationships or situations in the present relate to past experiences and in particular to childhood experiences. Throughout childhood we learn ways of relating to others and seeing the world. These ways of relating are carried with us into adulthood, often without conscious awareness. Of particular importance is what we learn about attachments to significant others, as this has implications for women in the attachments they will form with their babies during pregnancy and the postnatal period.

When an individual is unclear about why they are behaving, thinking or feeling a certain way, it is likely that unconscious processes are at play. Individuals may seek to hide difficult or unacceptable feelings using unconscious defence mechanisms. These mechanisms may have been learned in childhood and at that time served a useful purpose. However, in adulthood, they may no longer be necessary, but either the individual is not aware of these mechanisms or, if there is conscious awareness, the individual is finding it difficult to let go of them. In understanding this, the person becomes freer of anxieties and more in control of thoughts and feelings.

Two common defence mechanisms which are often referred to in day-to-day language are *projection* and *denial*.

Projection is used to describe a situation where individuals attribute their own undesirable feelings to someone else and, in doing so, avoid addressing the feeling in themselves. For example, the pregnant woman who is convinced her partner is uncertain about having a baby when in fact she is herself very ambivalent about the pregnancy/baby and becoming a mother.

Denial refers to a defence whereby individuals fail to see the reality of a situation and therefore keep themselves safe from having to deal with the emotional impact. A good example of this is someone in an abusive relationship who denies the abuse even though others can clearly see what is happening.

The work we do in therapy is to enable the patient to explore what are often very confusing feelings with a view to uncovering the unconscious processes at play. This may involve pointing out patterns of behaviour, making links with the past, identifying defences which may have been helpful but no longer serve a purpose, and could even be sabotaging of self and/or relationships. In doing this, the aim is to support women to become more aware and gain a greater understanding of themselves and to separate the past from the present.

Women for whom this model could be particularly helpful are those who present with:

- fear of being like their own mothers,
- fear of repeating abusive patterns from their own childhoods,
- fear of loss of identity,
- belief about themselves as 'not good enough' or bad,
- critical and judgemental thoughts about themselves or
- fear that they will damage their baby.

Sometimes women will not be able to articulate these concerns initially but will present as very anxious about the pregnancy or becoming a mother or feeling very low, angry or irritable. The work is to look below the surface to see what these feelings mean and how they might relate to the past.

Cognitive behavioural therapy approach

Cognitive behavioural therapy (CBT) is commonly used in the work we do with women. This type of therapy is more focussed on changing the way an individual thinks or behaves to better manage symptoms/problems. It is most

Box 3.4 Practice learning point

A woman may come to therapy feeling extremely confused about negative feelings towards the pregnancy, given that the pregnancy had been planned and wanted for some time. The work of therapy is to think about the reasons for this. These feelings may relate to the woman's own childhood experiences, the relationship with her own mother, ideas about herself and her body and the losses that are involved in becoming a mother.

commonly used to treat anxiety and depression but can be useful for other mental health issues as well as physical problems, such as pain management. We developed the use of CBT within the service as a response to women presenting with high levels of anxiety and depression who needed support with day-to-day functioning during pregnancy. Some women required support with strategies to manage a particular anxiety-provoking event, such as the birth of their baby or a medical procedure. CBT can also be helpful for women who are unable to use insight techniques (outlined in the section on psychodynamic approach); instead they can be helped with developing tools and strategies for managing psychological symptoms.

Box 3.5 Cognitive behavioural therapy techniques

- Challenging automatic negative thoughts
- Reframing these thoughts and finding alternative ways of thinking
- Relaxation, breathing exercises and mindfulness (Kabat-Zinn, 2004)
- Visualisation including safe place imagery (Scott, 2012; Scott & Stradling, 2006)
- Distraction
- Desensitisation
  - Breaking problems down into smaller more manageable areas

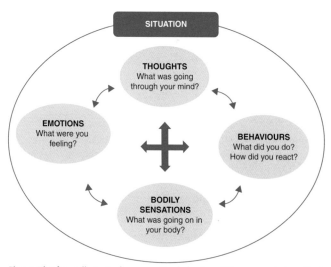

Fig 3.1 This figure illustrates how cognitive behavioural therapy can help patients to understand how thoughts, behaviours, bodily sensations and emotions interact in a given situation.

Box 3.6 Women for whom this model could be particularly helpful are those who present with:

- Anxiety
- Depression
- Sleep problems
- Somatisation
- Phobias

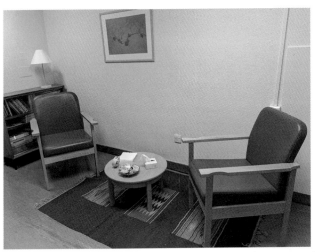

Fig 3.2 Image of a counselling room set-up prior to a consultation. Note the position of the clock on the table, to ensure the session is kept to time without interrupting the therapeutic flow.

Case studies

In the following section, we draw on the theoretical interventions given previously to present three case studies that demonstrate the work we undertake as part of the women's health counselling service. To protect patient confidentiality, the examples we have used are composite case studies based on a number of women who have attended our service. We hope to illustrate the themes that emerge in the psychological work we do with women.

Case study using a psychodynamic approach

D is a woman in her early 40s, originally from New Zealand. This was her first pregnancy. The pregnancy was planned and much wanted. She lived with her partner. She was referred to the women's health counselling service as she was experiencing anxiety, low mood and insomnia. She had experienced some anxiety and stress related to her work in the past. However, she was surprised to find herself feeling psychologically distressed at a time when she imagined she would feel excited and hopeful in her first pregnancy.

There were several strands to D's symptoms as we gradually explored her thoughts in the counselling sessions. It transpired that although she very much wanted a baby, she felt ambivalent about the huge change this would mean in her life. She felt guilty about acknowledging and expressing these feelings, as if by admitting them they would harm the baby and she would be punished. Her identity was bound up with her successful career, and she feared the loss of status and position that could result from maternity leave. The counselling aimed to normalise these thoughts, as, in fact, many women in her position have similar thoughts and feelings. In particular, acknowledging negative as well as positive feelings about the pregnancy helped D start to appreciate the complexity of her emotions and to come to terms with them. It was also important to explore that having thoughts and feelings did not mean they transform into reality and that it was beneficial to express them rather than act upon them. D felt that she would damage the baby psychologically by admitting she felt ambivalent. It emerged in the counselling that D's mother had given up her own career to look after her, and she had expressed some resentment and anger about having done this. D was consequently worried that she may have the same feelings towards her own child.

In the counselling sessions, it transpired that D had very high expectations of herself and was a perfectionist. She wanted to have the perfect natural birth and be the "best" mother to her child. She was inhabited by a highly critical and judgemental internal voice. She also liked to be in control. All of this was increasing her anxiety, low mood and insomnia. We explored the origins of her perfectionism and then looked at the underlying unconscious fears. She explained that both her parents had high expectations of her as a child. They wanted her to excel at school and were very critical of any failure. She had internalised these views, and they had become part of the way she perceived herself and the pressures she put on herself. She had not been aware of this, and she was then able to see how damaging this had been for her and could potentially be to her child if she repeated a similar pattern. It transpired that her perfectionism was a defence she used unconsciously to hide her fear of weakness, vulnerability and falling apart. These fears related to her mother who, during the whole of her childhood and teenage years, had suffered from various physical illnesses, had issues with mental health to

(Continued)

the extent of, at times, being an inpatient in a psychiatric hospital. For D, this meant she felt pressure to be strong and resilient, unable to share with others her fears or what she considered her weaknesses. This exacerbated her anxiety and added to the stress she placed on herself. It became apparent that she held an underlying fear of experiencing similar mental health problems to her mother, and she had to defend herself against this possibility by repressing such thoughts. Instead, these thoughts emerged as anxiety and low mood. In being able to consciously voice her thoughts and feelings openly in a safe and confidential setting, these fears became less powerful. She could begin to see that by acknowledging areas she perceived as a weakness or failure, she could be more open and intimate with her partner and friends and feel less alone. She saw that by expressing her vulnerability in the counselling sessions, she had not fallen apart or become mentally ill, and neither had her counsellor. This was especially important as it contrasted with her experience of her mother, who had been unable to cope in this way. D became aware that the way her mother experienced physical pain had affected her so that she had internalised a terror of such pain, which was then transferred onto her fears of how she would experience childbirth. Her mother had unconsciously instilled in her an idea that health professionals could not be trusted and that she would have to manage on her own.

D's anxiety and insomnia were also related to her partner and manifested themselves in irritation, annoyance and fear that he would not be able to respond to her expectations when the baby was born. She was often unable to sleep because of her dreams of being abandoned and left alone with a crying baby. In the counselling sessions, we explored how her feelings towards her partner were partly her own projections of her feelings about the transition to motherhood. In exploring her dreams of abandonment there appeared to be links with her sense that her infantile needs were not understood and responded to by her parents, as her mother was preoccupied with her physical and mental health and her father was busy working and left when she was 10 years old. She was then able to acknowledge that her present situation was very different from that of her parents. Her mother, she said, had been very critical of her father and very controlling around bringing her up. In contrast, she had a supportive partner who very much wanted to be fully involved with his child. She was then able to see that her own overly controlling and organising behaviour towards her partner and her irritation with him could potentially push him away and bring about her biggest fear of being abandoned again. She realised that she could potentially repeat a similar pattern of behaviour with her partner as her mother had with her father.

Case study using cognitive behavioural therapy approach

S is a woman in her mid-30s who was referred to us by her midwife towards the end of her second pregnancy. She was brought up in America and came from a family originally from China. She met her British husband in America, and they had recently moved to London, where he grew up, as he had organised a work transfer to a London office. They have one son, aged 3 years, who was born in America.

S was referred because she was terrified of giving birth again. She had recently been experiencing panic attacks, anxiety, terror and flashbacks. In the first counselling session, it transpired that the birth of her first child had been very traumatic. Her labour had not progressed, the baby's heartbeat suddenly dropped on the monitor and the obstetric team decided that she would have to have an emergency caesarean section (C-section). Her husband was not able to be with her in the theatre. She explained that the epidural did not completely work, and she experienced excruciating pain when the C-section was performed. She could recall the feeling she had when the surgeon made the incision. She said she had been deeply affected by this at the time, but the physical and emotional demands of her baby and the passage of time had lessened the memories of her birth experience and she had not thought about it during the last few years. As she neared the birth of her second baby, these memories had emerged in flashbacks and were making her feel anxious and in a state of panic. She had been told by her consultant that due to her previous birth experience she would need to have a planned C-section.

After an initial consultation for counselling, it was decided with S that a CBT approach would be beneficial given the nature of her psychological presentation and the fact that she was due to give birth in less than 2 months. We agreed that it would be helpful to have several strategies she could practice at home before birth and during birth. These CBT strategies included exploring her thoughts and finding alternative thoughts, distraction, relaxation, breathing methods and visualisation. The strategies also addressed improving communication with her husband and the multi-disciplinary team in the hospital.

Thoughts: We explored S's thoughts regarding her previous birth and the imminent birth of her second baby. Her mind was dominated by negative and catastrophic ideas. Her thoughts fluctuated between imagining that the epidural would not work, that she would feel the extreme pain of the surgeon's instrument cutting her open, bleeding to death, having a panic attack during the C-section, screaming in pain and that she would be unable to control her anxiety. One of the main

(Continued)

methods of CBT is to help patients become aware of how their negative automatic thoughts/catastrophic thinking affect their emotions, their somatic state and their behaviour. This way of thinking and its impact on the patient can become a vicious cycle of constant negativity and have consequences for all aspects of the patient's functioning. To change this, it is necessary to adjust the original thoughts and reframe them in a more positive and less persecutory way. We were able to identify S's negative thoughts and how they increased anxiety and panic, leading her to feel physically unwell with headaches and stomach pain. This produced impatient and irritable behaviour towards her husband and child and an inability to complete tasks around the home. In the counselling sessions, S examined whether there was evidence for such negative thinking in this different situation. She was then able to challenge her negative thoughts and replace them with different and less persecutory ones. She was able to acknowledge that the situation was very different from her previous experience. The C-section was planned this time, which meant she could prepare for it. The consultant, anaesthetist and midwives were fully aware of what had happened during her first birth and would ensure that the epidural was working effectively. She had built up a good and trusting relationship with her midwife and medical staff. She knew that it was not in the interest of the medical staff to allow her to die and that everything would be done to ensure the safety of her and the baby.

Distraction: We discussed ways she could distract herself when the disturbing and anxious thoughts occurred. She identified a number of activities she enjoyed and potentially could be helpful, such as watching a film in the evening with her husband, listening to calming music, performing household tasks like cleaning, playing with her 3-year-old, going for a walk and attending yoga classes.

Relaxation, breathing and mindfulness: There is now much evidence to show that relaxation, breathing and mindfulness (Kabat-Zinn, 2004) is beneficial in reducing stress, panic and anxiety. These techniques have an impact on the neurological pathways of the brain, releasing chemicals such as endorphins that elevate mood and can influence self-esteem and resilience (Coleman & Davidson, 2018).

In the counselling session, we practised breathing techniques that enabled S to concentrate on her breath and where the breath was in her body. We also worked on ways of acknowledging the thoughts in her mind but not engaging with them, instead letting them go.

S was encouraged to practise these techniques every day for about 20 minutes if possible, in a quiet place where she would not be interrupted. If she experienced panic attacks or anxiety, she was to use this method of controlling her breathing.

Visualisation: This technique is used a lot with patients who are experiencing post traumatic stress disorder, and there are claims that it is effective (Scott, 2012; Scott & Stradling, 2006). S was experiencing vivid flashbacks of her previous C-section that were preventing her from sleeping at night and exacerbating the anxiety and panic. She was particularly worried that during the C-section she would have one of her flashbacks and that this would produce a severe panic attack and something terrible would happen. We explored a scene that she could conjure up in her mind, one that she found calming and peaceful and could take herself to when the flashback occurred. S visualised a scene from her childhood of a place she had spent holidays with her family, a lake surrounded by mountains and trees, blue skies and warm sun – a place associated with happy memories. As part of this technique, when the flashback occurred, she was told to imagine placing the memory in a box and locking it with a key and then to take her mind to the calmer place she had chosen. This technique requires practise for the patient to be familiar and comfortable, and S was advised to practise each day.

Communication: Another helpful element was encouraging S to clearly communicate her experience, her psychological state and her fears to the multi-disciplinary team. This enabled her to build a more trusting relationship with the team, which had an impact on her psychological state. The counselling sessions helped her to articulate her concerns and think about ways of communicating them to the team. This enabled her to feel more in control of her maternity care and birth experience. She also built up an open and trusting communication with her midwife. Visiting and familiarising herself with the labour ward was helpful as her previous experience of birth was in America where health care, she said, was very different. Her anxiety and sense of not feeling in control was also, in part, exacerbated by her lack of knowledge of the National Health Service (NHS) and maternity services in the United Kingdom. The counselling also included familiarising her with the system here. She was also encouraged to share the strategies we had discussed with her husband so that he could help her to practise them at home and remind her during the birth if she became anxious and frightened or experienced a flashback.

Case study using a psychodynamic approach with cognitive behavioural therapy elements

G is a woman in her late 20s who was referred by her midwife to the women's health counselling service during her second pregnancy. She presented with extreme anxiety that was having an impact on her day-to-day life. She was struggling to get to work and avoiding most social situations.

At the first appointment, G reported that much of the anxiety was focussed on the pregnancy and the wellbeing of her baby. She was frequently searching the internet for information to check that any symptoms she experienced were 'normal'. She was also tracking the baby's movements to the extent that she found it hard to concentrate on other things and hard to sleep, as she churned over thoughts about the health of her baby.

G was aware that much of this anxiety related to having experienced a stillbirth at 34 weeks of pregnancy the previous year. She felt that with this second pregnancy she had to be 'watchful' in case she missed a sign of something wrong.

We agreed to meet for regular sessions with a goal of learning cognitive behavioural therapy (CBT) based tools for managing anxiety day to day whilst also giving time to the loss of her first baby and preparation for this baby.

Much of the early sessions focussed on managing the anxiety. We talked about G's fears and need to be 'watchful' and began to identify when her thoughts were helpful and when they tipped into being unhelpful. Thinking is helpful for problem-solving but becomes unhelpful when the thoughts churn, looking for a solution as a response to the unbearable nature of uncertainty.

It emerged that G had experienced a very chaotic childhood. She was well cared for in material terms and could recall some very happy memories of birthdays and holidays. However, her father 'had a temper' and the family lived with a sense that at any time his temper could flare up. The worst times were when he would be so angry he would shout at their mother and lash out at her. The anger wasn't usually directed at G or her siblings (she had two older sisters), but they witnessed and heard these events. She recalled being scared and confused at these times. We began to understand that G had responded to the uncertainty of childhood by finding comfort and safety in structure, planning and routine. Her first pregnancy was planned; she had ideas of how it would be and plans for when her baby was born. When it didn't work out that way, G was thrown back to feelings of fear and confusion. To manage these feelings, she was anxiously searching for certainty again on the internet and by tracking her baby's movements.

Alongside this psychodynamic understanding, whereby we linked past with present experience, we talked about measures for managing day-to-day life. G began to feel able to restrict her internet searches once she had identified that they triggered unhelpful thinking. We talked about distraction techniques in the form of things she enjoyed doing, and she decided she could go for a walk or phone a friend when she noticed her thoughts spiralling.

It was interesting when we talked more about the pregnancy that, although G was very focussed on signs of the baby being okay, she found it very hard to actually envisage the baby or to think about her being born. In fact, in the very early weeks of pregnancy, she had refused to even think of herself as pregnant. We were able to begin to compare this recent response to her response towards the previous pregnancy and understand that G was protecting herself from further loss by not bonding with this baby. The flip side was she felt very guilty about this.

Feelings of guilt were dominant throughout the sessions. G felt guilty that her first baby (R) had died, and felt that in some way it must have been her fault. She had lots of 'what if' thoughts that often amounted to 'what if I had done something differently'. She felt guilty for not thinking enough about her second baby while also feeling disloyal to R if she did.

We were able to explore how hard it was for her to have two babies in mind. She said, 'That would be easy if they were both alive,' which enabled us to talk about how hard it is to know how to think about a baby who has died. Until the second pregnancy, G had taken a 'just get on with it' approach and had tried not to think about R too much, but this defence mechanism was no longer working. Alongside feelings of guilt, she was angry and sad. She found herself getting angry with her sister for not mentioning R enough. On exploration, we were able to see that perhaps her sister received some anger that didn't belong to her but rather belonged to the situation and maybe to herself for her own 'forgetting' of R when she thought about this new pregnancy.

During the middle stage of sessions, much of the focus was on R and how to remember her. As we approached the anniversary of her birth, G wondered about how to commemorate her. We talked about the importance of rituals and how, for many life events, we know what rituals are appropriate. G said, 'No one tells you what to do when your baby has died'. In discussion with her partner, G decided she wanted to visit the cemetery on the anniversary of R's death. G also began to think about R's place in the home and with her wider family. She didn't want her to be forgotten and decided to have a necklace made and to have a photo of her handprint to sit alongside the other family photos.

(Continued)

As G began to find a clearer place for R in her mind and in her home/ family, she was able to turn her thoughts more to the idea of having a live baby. She was very tentative about this at first, not being able to trust that all would be well, but she did begin to have an image of herself with this baby in her mind.

However, each week G continued to recount how the current pregnancy was progressing, the anxiety she had experienced during the week and her continuing thoughts about the safety of this pregnancy. She was using the techniques we had talked about, limiting her internet searches and distracting herself, but sometimes she felt overwhelmed with fear and would experience a feeling of panic. To address this, we explored the idea of safe place imagery, a visualisation technique described in the previous case.

In the final stages of counselling, G began to talk about being a mother and the very confusing ideas she had about whether she (and others) thought she was already a mother or not. She had ideas about what kind of mother she wanted to be and she felt that R dying proved she was not the mother she had wanted to be. This had left her feeling she was a bad mother who was not attentive enough and was unable to protect her baby.

Thoughts began to emerge about her own experience of being mothered. She described her own mother as being very caring and attentive much of the time but also described an unpredictable quality that often left her uncertain of her mother's attention. As an adult, G could surmise that because her mother was experiencing domestic violence, there were times when her thoughts were elsewhere, but as a child G didn't have this understanding and simply felt abandoned and unprotected. We were able to see that G had been determined not to be like her mother in this respect, and R's death had left her feeling that, like her own mother, she wasn't able to protect her baby. Being able to make the connection between her own childhood experiences and her current thoughts and feelings enabled G to understand them better and ultimately not to be so tortured by them.

As the counselling came to an end, whilst still anxious, G was able to think about the coming birth, to prepare at home for the baby's arrival and to have a more measured view of what the outcome might be.

In conclusion, G presented with severe anxiety which needed to be addressed and managed to enable her to function better day to day. However, we were able to explore the underlying cause of anxiety in terms of the recent loss and its meaning for her, given her own early experiences. As the work progressed, G was able to move focus from R to the new baby and ultimately found that it was possible to have both of her babies in her mind.

Quantitative evaluation

The service we provide is evaluated using both quantitative and qualitative methods. Our quantitative data are collected via the CORE system (Clinical Outcomes in Routine Evaluation), for which patients fill in a 10-point questionnaire to measure distress at the beginning and end of treatment. Scores are compared with national cut-off scores, established by comparing scores of those who report mental health problems with those who do not. If distress scores show a decrease from start to end of counselling, we may deduce that our treatment has been effective. Over a number of years, results have consistently shown a decrease in levels of distress for the majority of the women we see.

As well as evaluating the service, there are other advantages to filling in these questionnaires. Some of the women we see will be totally unfamiliar with the idea of counselling and can feel uncomfortable in this new arena. Completing the questionnaire with women at their first session provides a structure for them to begin to tell us about themselves and how life is for them.

In addition, one of the questions relates to suicidal thoughts and actions. This can be a good way of introducing the topic of risk to help us to assess whether the woman needs any immediate support to stay safe. Filling in the questionnaire again as we come to the end of counselling is helpful for many women to review the experience and assess if and how there has been change.

More information about this system of evaluation and a copy of the CORE-10 questionnaire can be found at https://www.coreims.co.uk.

Qualitative evaluation

In addition to using the CORE-10 data to assess the degree of psychological change from the start to the end of the counselling, it is useful to employ qualitative research methods to gain a more in-depth understanding of the experience and how valuable the counselling service is for women. For instance, we asked MSc student Abigail Enlander to develop a questionnaire to collate the opinions of the women we see. Questions included the appropriateness of the setting, waiting times and general satisfaction with the counselling service (Enlander, 2017). Women were given these questionnaires in their penultimate counselling session. Most of the answers to the questions demonstrated that our counselling service was highly valued and appreciated by the patients. Women stated that they felt listened to and that their concerns were taken seriously. Feedback from women also suggested that the relationship with their counsellor was crucial in enabling them to address their issues and move forward psychologically.

> 'One potential reason that counsellors at the women's health counselling service were perceived to be so beneficial was because of the way they were able to help women move from their lowest point into a more positive frame of mind' (Enlander, 2017, p. 21). Comments from patients included 'I would be in a terrible place if (counsellor) was not here, life would be very difficult. This has pulled me out of a very dark place', 'I feel more positive and hopeful', 'counselling played a very big role in my gaining the courage to live and persevere' (Ibid.).

Some women's feedback highlighted several areas that were helpful for the service to consider in terms of improvement. These included the limitation of the number of counselling sessions. Several women felt they would have liked more sessions as it took time to engage with counselling. The counselling room was felt to be comfortable by most patients but for some who had lost a baby it was painful to come to a room on the maternity floor. Overall, the main therapeutic model of psychodynamic counselling was helpful to most of the women but there were some who would have liked more 'tools' and strategies to manage their concerns. This latter finding was particularly useful in confirming to us that it was important to offer an eclectic therapeutic approach including psychodynamic, CBT and mindfulness interventions. It also highlighted that, during the initial counselling consultation, it is important to assess which therapeutic approach or combination would be most beneficial for each woman, particularly given the constraints of short-term therapy.

The multi-disciplinary team

There are many advantages to working in a multi-disciplinary team (MDT) when considering how to develop a service sensitive to the psychological needs of pregnant women. In our own working context, the women's health counselling service is part of the multi-disciplinary maternity team in a large

Box 3.7 Practice learning point

Examples of MDT discussions

A woman who is refusing to have an internal examination and becomes tearful or angry about this may well have a history of being sexually abused.

Women who insist on having a caesarean section may have had a previous traumatic birth or a history of sexual abuse.

Anxious women may find the hospital frightening due to previous negative experiences of hospital admissions.

National Health Service (NHS) foundation trust based in a hospital setting. This location has enhanced the possibilities of providing a holistic service to patients to include their medical, psychological and educational needs. To do this effectively, it is important that there is thoughtful, reflective and respectful communication between all the professionals. As counsellors, we take an active part in MDT meetings including the psychosocial meetings where vulnerable women and those with safeguarding concerns are discussed. We also attend the specialist perinatal mental health team meetings. Outside these meetings, we liaise with midwives, doctors and physiotherapists within the hospital and externally with other agencies, which include social care, psychiatric/psychological services, general practitioners (GPs), solace women's aid and children and family centres. Our role is to ensure that members of the MDT are aware of and understand the psychological history of women and how this might affect their clinical presentation. This will help guide the MDT in their communication with these women.

Equally, it is helpful for us as counsellors to understand the medical health and physical issues of the women we see during pregnancy to understand how these have an impact on their psychological state.

Supervision and reflective groups for midwives

All health professionals require opportunities to think about their work to process the emotional demands and to share best practice, furthermore it is well documented that midwives (as well as nurses) suffer with burnout and stress (Kinman, Teoh, & Hariss, 2020). As counsellors, we are required by our training organisations to have regular individual supervision. We also have organised reflective practice meetings within the hospital and with other counsellors from a different department, as well as holding our own peer supervision.

We offer a reflective space to the bereavement midwives and have run a group for staff on the postnatal ward to help them think about their work. It is important for both professional and personal development that midwives are offered a space to register and reflect on feelings and thoughts that may occur during interactions with women or difficult clinical scenarios. This may include managing excessive clinical workloads and caring for women who are emotionally distressed.

There are a number of ways in which the sessions described above can benefit the psychological and physical wellbeing of midwives.

Exploring the depth of reaction to work situations may help midwives to understand more about their own behaviours such as poor communication with patients, taking stress home and overeating or drinking. In turn it can enable them to think about self-care such as taking breaks, regular meals and exercise as an alternative. The importance of rest and relaxation time can be highlighted in the group, and midwives can be signposted to easily available relaxation and mindfulness apps and internet information.

A greater understanding of the impact of the work on oneself can also enable midwives to better support each other by noticing what is happening for colleagues during a demanding shift or challenging clinical scenario and actively providing help.

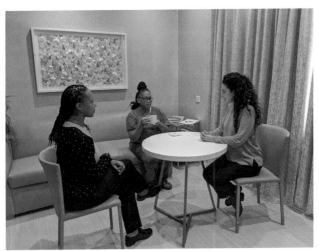

Fig 3.3 Reflective group session for midwives.

Box 3.8 Reflection on burnout in midwifery

Stephanie, midwife for Acacia Team (vulnerable women)
Barnet Hospital

Burnout is very real for all those working in health care. This can be magnified when specialising in a midwifery role, especially in a team supporting vulnerable women. In addition to standard midwifery care, there is extra training, referrals, multi-professional working, child protection/child in need meetings, and the enhanced pathway of care to provide. Working late regularly in a team with such emotionally dependent women is physically and emotionally draining.

  This is why self-care is important, including making a conscious effort to finish on time, mindfully leaving cases at work and clearing your mind. Additionally, it makes a difference for days off to truly be days off and for rest to be a priority. Easy to say and not so easy to do – I am still working on it.

It is also important for midwives' psychological wellbeing that they feel able to provide feedback to managers, either in the relevant meetings or individually, about concerns over work or personal issues rather than feeling that they have to cope on their own. The reflective group can support them in doing this.

If the psychological stresses are ones which midwives are unable to manage on their own, there are a number of counselling and psychological services they can confidentially refer themselves to either through the hospital, privately or through their GP, and the group can act as a reminder of these resources.

Conclusion

In this chapter we have given an introduction to some of the psychological concerns that can impact the relationship between mother and baby and illustrated how these can be addressed in counselling. Enabling the mother to gain a greater understanding of her thoughts and feelings during this crucial time can influence the relationship long term and in turn influence the baby's future relationships.

We have highlighted the importance of good communication and sharing within the multi-disciplinary team so that the patient's needs are thought about. The staff reflective groups and our own supervision are integral firstly to enhancing a better understanding of the psychological concerns facing mothers and secondly enabling us, as professionals, to be aware of our own personal psychological responses to our patients.

POINTS FOR REFLECTION

- In this chapter, you have been introduced to a psychodynamic under-standing of women's responses to present day situations. How might this influence your thinking in a challenging situation with a woman?
- In this chapter, you have been given information about a number of CBT techniques. Which of these do you think might be most helpful to women you see?
- In this chapter, we have highlighted the importance of self-care for midwives. Can you think of one change you could make to your life-style that might reflect better self-care?

References

Bowlby, J. (1969). *Attachment and loss volume 1: Attachment*. Harmondsworth: Penguin.

Coleman, D., & Davidson, R. J. (2018). *The science of meditation, how to change your brain, mind and body*. Harmondsworth: Penguin.

Enlander, A. (2017). *The women's health counselling service: Helping women to "gain the courage to live and persevere" after mental health difficulties in the perinatal period. (Master's thesis)*. Anna Freud Centre/UCL.

Greenberger, D., & Padesky, C. (1995). *Mind over mood*. New York: Guilford Press.

Kabat-Zinn, J. (2004). *Wherever you go, there you are: Mindfulness meditation for everyday life*. London: Piatkus.

Kinman, G., Teoh, K., & Hariss, A. (2020). *The mental health & wellbeing of nurses & midwives in the United Kingdom*. The Society of Occupational Medicine. https://documentcloud.adobe.com/link/track?uri=urn:aaid:scds:US:6613f-d8a-031b-4f48-9ddc-f2448a1113f5#pageNum=68.

Klein, M. (1940). Mourning and its relation to manic-depressive states. *International Journal of Psycho-Analysis, 21*, 125–153.

Perinatal Mental Health Services for London. (2017). *Guide for Commissioners*. Healthy London Partnership/Clinical Network NHS England London Region.

Scott, M. (2012). *CBT for common trauma*. London: Sage.

Scott, M., & Stradling, S. (2006). *Counselling for post traumatic stress disorders*. London: Sage.

Spurling, L. (2004). *An introduction to psychodynamic counselling*. London: Palgrave.

Westbrook, D., Kennedy, H., & Kirk, J. (2007). *An introduction to cognitive behaviour therapy, skills and applications*. London: Sage.

Winnicott, D. W. (1973). *The child, the family and the outside world*. Harmondsworth: Penguin.

Web resources

The CORE Outcome Measure (CORE-OM) [online] available at: http://www.coreims.co.uk/About_Core_System_Outcome_Measure.html. Accessed 10 September 2020.

Headspace: https://www.headspace.com

NHS: https://www.nhs.uk/conditions/stress-anxiety-depression/mindfulnes

Oxford Cognitive Therapy Centre: https://www.octc.co.uk/resources

Public Health England. (2019). *Guidance 4. Perinatal Mental Health*. https://www.gov.uk/government/publications/better-mental-health-jsna-toolkit/4-perinatal-mental-health. Accessed 16 August 2020.

CHAPTER 4

Complex social factors

Kate Clements and Tania Staras

Introduction

Midwives and midwifery have a clear public profile in the UK – most people think they know what a midwife does. Midwives see women antenatally and postnatally, but most importantly in the public mind, they deliver babies. However, the role of the midwife is multi-faceted and extends far beyond this perceived stereotypical image. Midwives are skilled, autonomous professionals who support the complexity of women's lives throughout the childbearing year. Some of the most significant and challenging complexities include issues relating to mental and psychological health and illness, in particular those situations where there are a range of factors involved.

This chapter begins to put mental health into a broader context by considering conditions and situations that may be cause and effect of psychological need or distress. These areas can be challenging for midwives, particularly if they do not feel that they have specialist knowledge and expertise. Peoples' lives can be incredibly complex with issues of housing, financial need, social issues and mental health compounding the state of pregnancy. For some women, the pregnancy may almost seem secondary to their other stresses and needs.

Some of the issues that midwives may see in practice include domestic abuse, modern slavery and substance misuse. They are, however, not the only complex social and psychological issues that midwives may come across while caring for women and their families. Not all issues will be experienced equally; for some people, these issues will lead to significant psychological distress and for others much less so. Similarly, situations are not always linear. Substance misuse may, for example, be both cause and effect of mental distress. Similarly, factors may not be seen in isolation; for example, sexual abuse may result in both substance misuse and perinatal mental health issues. This chapter uses case study and discussion alongside current resources to explore the mental health aspects and to allow midwives to see their role in practical focus. The ideas and approaches outlined can be adapted to be applicable across a range of areas.

Table 4.1 highlights some of the principles of caregiving in complex situations.

Table 4.1: Principles of midwifery care for complex social factors

Tackling stigma	Being non-judgemental, valuing individuals
Lifelong learning	Self-directed learning study days to ensure an up-to-date understanding of issues and care
Supporting emotional and physical wellbeing	Providing core midwifery roles. Seeing the woman as a whole person, not just a 'problem'
Signposting and referral	Understanding and using care pathways and specialist services; working with others
Building trust	Demonstrating kindness and compassion; working alongside women
Identifying risk	Understanding the significance of changing situations and pressure points; working with women and other agencies to mitigate risk
Working with families	Supporting the whole family; where appropriate, using specialist support

The role of the specialist midwife

Traditionally midwives were expected to be able to offer care across the whole childbearing year, working in different settings. They are still seen as the experts and lead caregivers in all aspects of normal pregnancy, birth and the postnatal period. However, over the last 20 years a range of factors has impacted on these core midwifery roles. These include an increasingly complex childbearing population, with age, obesity and co-morbidities affecting care delivery. There has also been a recognition of the impact of wider social and psychological issues on pregnancy and birth and the need to support and mitigate these in an appropriate way. These concerns have in turn led to the growth of specialist midwifery roles to support groups considered vulnerable or at risk (Royal College of Midwives (RCM), 2013). One of the aims of specialist roles is to keep women from falling through the gaps in services, such as between maternity and mental health services. The roles are variable both in coverage and scope; some trusts will have a range of specialists, and others far fewer. They foreground the role of the midwife in public health but tend to be quite vulnerable to changes in funding streams and health service priorities. Some areas have developed a range of specialist roles only to have to merge or cut them due to budgetary constraints. *Table 4.2 gives an overview of the variety of responsibilities which may fall to the specialist midwife.'*

Table 4.2: **The role of the specialist midwife**

Expert care	May provide clinical care to a group of women or caseload
Working across professions	May include developing care plans, attending case conferences; working with social services and other agencies
Development of guidelines/ research	Takes a lead in developing evidence-based guidelines to support care for specialist services. This may also involve developing and implementing research projects
Care pathways and integration	Develops care pathways that are used across the service, including by those in non-specialist roles. Ensures that care is integrated and not fragmented
Education and training	Supports the education and training of the multi-disciplinary team, including midwives, doctors, students, support workers and allied services such as paramedics
Quality improvement/clinical governance	Provides expert input and leadership to ensure care is up-to-date and follows best practice
Advice	Formal and informal advice and support to caregivers and health professionals in non-specialist roles
Champions	Advocates for patients and champions the issue across a range of platforms. Works to remove stigma and develop understanding and appropriate care

Domestic abuse

Background and definitions

In 2013 a national definition of domestic abuse was agreed on that brings together all the possible elements of the issue. The definition is wide-ranging and reminds us that abuse can manifest in many ways, and these can change over time:

> *Any incident or pattern of incidents of controlling, coercive or threatening behaviour, violence or violence between those aged 16 or over who are or have been intimate partners or family members regardless of gender or sexuality. This can encompass, but is not limited to, the following types of violence: psychological; physical; sexual; financial; emotional.*

> *Controlling behaviour is: a range of acts designed to make a person subordinate and/or dependent by isolating them from sources of support, exploiting their resources and capacities for personal gain, depriving them of the means needed for independence, resistance and escape*

and regulating their everyday behaviour. Coercive behaviour is: an act or a pattern of acts of assault, threats, humiliation and intimidation or other violence that is used to harm, punish, or frighten their victim. (HM Govt, 2013).

It is also recognised that abuse can begin, escalate or change during pregnancy. Because pregnancy is a time when women have sustained and regular contact with the health services, it may be the first time that patterns of behaviour or injury are recognised. There is an expectation that midwives will ask about abuse and violence during routine antenatal and postnatal encounters. This should be done when the woman is alone with the health professional. If interpreting services are required, these should be via a professional rather than through informal arrangements such as family or friends. There are note-making conventions that allow responses to be discreetly documented in a way which cannot be picked up by perpetrators. Approximately 80% of women experiencing domestic abuse seek help from health services and these are often a woman's first, or only, point of contact (National Institute of Clinical Excellence (NICE), 2020; Webb et al., 2020).

Practice learning point

This scenario relates to a woman being the alleged victim of abuse, which is more commonplace in a maternity setting as the pregnant woman is the patient. However, it is important to consider that people of any gender can perpetrate domestic violence and abuse, and it can happen in different- and same-sex couples. Sometimes it is unclear whether a mother or mother-to-be is the victim or perpetrator of abuse. Physical abuse perpetrated by a woman against a man may not always be perceived in the same way as it would if it was the other way round. Some men may also hold this view and therefore do not identify themselves as victims of domestic abuse. Health professionals need to remain alert to children living in a family where domestic abuse is being perpetrated by a woman and not underestimate the risk this could pose (NSPCC, 2020).

Managing the case study

Sara has disclosed information about the nature of her injuries and then retracted this. This is not uncommon; women may want professionals to know but at the same time be very anxious about the consequences of sharing information. There is a concern in this scenario that the woman has a changing story and may be minimising what has happened. This might be because of her own low self-esteem and also perhaps due to concerns about social services' involvement and the fear of having her children removed. This anxiety can have a significant effect on what women choose to disclose and to whom. Finally, Sara is likely to be anxious about the perpetrator of abuse finding out that she has attended for care; this in turn may escalate the violence.

It is important for midwives to be aware that domestic abuse can continue after parents have separated and sometimes the stress of separation can be a trigger for violent/abusive episodes among (previously) intimate partners. In this situation, professionals may underestimate the risk to children during relationship breakdown and disputes about post-separation contact. In addition, some domestic abuse relationships are characterised by separations and reconciliations. Professionals must be alert to the possibility that a separated couple may be back together and should not rely on a previous claim that the relationship had permanently ended (NSPCC, 2020).

When considering Sara's situation, it is also vital to bear in mind that domestic abuse does not discriminate; your background, your education, your wealth, your age, your job, where you grew up – none of it matters. The fact that the woman is a teacher does not mean that the situation should be approached any differently. In exploring the issue of domestic abuse in pregnancy, it is vital that health professionals avoid stereotypes and remain alert to possible abuse in all social and domestic situations.

Supporting Sara

All midwives faced with a situation such as Sara's need to bear in mind the core principles of validation, risk assessment, referral and record-keeping.

- **Validate:** If there is a positive disclosure, validate the experience with phrases like 'I believe you' or 'this is not your fault'. Support and reassure them that they are not alone and that there is help available. It is important to not advise victims to leave their partner/abuser as this may place them at further risk of harm without appropriate safety planning.
- **Risk assess:** Ask if the victim feels unsafe; if the reply is 'yes', see whether the person has a safe place to go (e.g. going to stay with a friend or family member). Consider admitting to the ward, if the victim agrees. If there are also children in the home, make an immediate safeguarding referral. Always discuss referrals with the victim as this can be a source of significant anxiety. In this scenario, even though Sara has not disclosed who the perpetrator is, a referral to children's social care should still be completed as Sara has experienced harm and her son could also be at risk of harm.
- **Action/refer:** Ask what support the victim has and what support might be needed. This may include referral to specialist midwifery support if available in your area. In this scenario the older child is 2 years old, so contact can be made with the allocated health visitor to see if they have identified any support needs or concerns for the

family. Some victims may feel ready to disclose to the police service. Refer to the independent and sexual violence advisor (IDSVA) with consent. Please see the role of the IDSVA below.

+ **Record-keeping:** Clearly document the situation and what actions have been taken (but make sure this is not in a place that the perpetrator can see, placing the person at greater risk of harm). There will be local conventions for recording and following up disclosure and actions; make sure you know what these are. (The list above is adapted from Pathfinder Toolkit – Webb et al., 2020.)

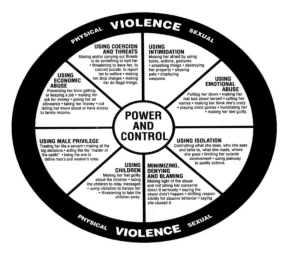

Fig 4.1 Dynamics of domestic violence and abuse. (https://www.theduluth model.org/wheels.)

The wheel above (fig. 4.1) reminds us of the complex and multi-faceted nature of abuse. It can be used by health professionals when talking to women. Women can point to each of the tactics on the wheel and clearly explain how these behaviours were used against them.

Domestic abuse and mental health

Domestic abuse can have an enormous effect on a person's mental health. It is now well accepted that abuse (both in childhood and in adult life) is often the main factor in the development of depression, anxiety and other mental health disorders and may lead to sleep disturbances, self-harm, suicide and attempted suicide, eating disorders and substance misuse. It is important to consider that if a person has a mental health illness/diagnosis, this may be used to abuse the person further. The victim may be in a particularly vulnerable position and may find it even harder to report domestic violence than another person without a mental health condition. The victim may also suffer from a sense of shame because of the stigma attached to having mental health diagnosis of any kind, which may make them feel even more powerless (Women's Aid, 2019).

If a woman presents to maternity services and reports that she is suffering from a mental health illness, it is important to identify whether there are any underlying factors such as domestic abuse that are affecting her mental health and emotional wellbeing.

Domestic abuse and midwives

Domestic abuse disclosure can be challenging for midwives to manage because of its complexity. Many midwives are anxious about saying or doing the wrong thing and thereby making the situation worse or feeling that they cannot do enough to support women. In these situations, it is vital to remember that support and information is available both from managers and from specialist services, as highlighted in the introduction to this chapter.

However, there may be another more personal aspect to domestic abuse for midwives; they may themselves be abuse survivors or currently living with abuse. This issue was explored in a 2018 RCM survey that highlighted the need for counselling and support services to be available to health professionals as well as members of the public (RCM, 2018). If you are concerned about your own situation or that of a colleague, then it is important to be aware that there is support available.

Female genital mutilation

Depending on the geographic area of work, midwives may encounter cases of female genital mutilation (FGM) quite frequently, occasionally or never. As with other complex social issues, unfamiliarity with a situation can make us uncomfortable and anxious about both recognising situations and giving appropriate advice, support and care. The World Health Organization (WHO) has developed definitions of types of FGM to help in clinical recognition (WHO, 2018) *see Table 4.3*. It states that FGM comprises all procedures that involve partial or total removal of the external female genitalia or other injury to the female genital organs for non-medical reasons.

Table 4.3: The WHO definition of female genital mutilation

Female genital mutilation is classified into 4 major types	Description
Type 1	The partial or total removal of the clitoral glans (the external and visible part of the clitoris, which is a sensitive part of the female genitals) and/or the prepuce/clitoral hood (the fold of skin surrounding the clitoral glans)
Type 2	The partial or total removal of the clitoral glans and the labia minora (the inner folds of the vulva), with or without removal of the labia majora (the outer folds of skin of the vulva)
Type 3	Also known as infibulation, this is the narrowing of the vaginal opening through the creation of a covering seal. The seal is formed by cutting and repositioning the labia minora, or labia majora, sometimes through stitching, with or without removal of the clitoral prepuce/clitoral hood and glans (type 1 female genital mutilation)
Type 4	This includes all other harmful procedures to the female genitalia for non-medical purposes (e.g. pricking, piercing, incising, scraping and cauterizing the genital area)

Adapted from World Health Organization (2018) Female genital mutilation [online] https://www.who.int/news-room/fact-sheets/detail/female-genital-mutilation

FGM is recognized internationally as a violation of the human rights of girls and women. It reflects deep-rooted inequality between the sexes and constitutes an extreme form of discrimination against women. It is nearly always carried out on minors and is a violation of the rights of children. The practice also violates a person's rights to health, security and physical integrity; the right to be free from torture and cruel, inhuman or degrading treatment and the right to life when the procedure results in death. It can result in mental health trauma, both in the short term and in the longer term as it impacts sexual health and relationships as well as self-image and self-esteem.

There is mandatory reporting of FGM in the UK (Department of Health (DH), 2016) where the procedure is illegal. Training is available to support health professionals in recognising the various types of procedure and the impact that these can have on reproductive health and childbirth. It is important to consider that some women may not be aware that they have had FGM; it might have happened when they were very young or be so prevalent in their community that they may not be aware of what unmutilated genitalia look like. Therefore, as in all areas of social complexity, it is important for midwives to be clear and unambiguous in communication. The following case study explores these ideas in practice.

Case Study 4.2

Bilan who is gravida 1 P0 attends the hospital at 39+2 weeks' gestation for a planned caesarean section as her unborn baby (female) is in a breech position. Bilan has had an unsuccessful external cephalic version (which is a process by which a breech baby can sometimes be turned from buttocks or foot first to head first) which was performed at 37 weeks.

Following completion of the relevant pre-operative checks, you take Bilan and her husband down to the theatre. In preparation for the surgery, you prepare to catheterise Bilan with her informed consent. On inspection the external genitalia appear abnormal and the catheterisation is difficult. Following discussion with the midwife in charge, it is found that the woman has had type 1 FGM.

This has not been disclosed at booking when the woman was previously screened.

Managing the case study

This scenario demonstrates that even with screening it is possible for women to go through their entire pregnancy without FGM being identified, especially if the woman is unaware that FGM ever took place. It is vital to communicate in a way that explores the issue without apportioning blame. It is also important to consider the potential adverse impact on Bilan's mental health.

Areas to consider in discussion include the following:

- Sensitively explore with the woman whether she comes from a community that practises cutting and whether she has knowledge of the procedure being performed. Is her husband aware? A family history of FGM is relevant for safeguarding.
- Take into account how the woman may feel when she finds out that she has had FGM and when she is informed that in the UK this is considered a form of abuse and that this may have been organised and undertaken by a family member/member of the community. Also consider how the woman may feel when she discusses FGM with fellow women within her community after being told about laws in the UK.
- Screen whether the woman has had any physical or psychological effect as a result of this being performed and refer appropriately for support if needed.

- Carry out risk assessment to help decide what steps to take using local or DH safeguarding guidance.
- Ensure that it is clearly documented on the woman's discharge summary that the woman has had FGM and that the health visitor and GP receive a copy of this following birth. It should also be clearly documented in the personal child health record (baby's red book).

Given that FGM is illegal in the UK, it is important to understand whether Bilan is aware of FGM in her wider community. If she, or any member of her family or community, plan for any female in the family to undergo FGM, then local safeguarding procedures should be followed and a referral made to children's services. Bilan should be given a copy of the *Statement Opposing Female Genital Mutilation* (HM Government, 2021), also known as the *FGM Health Passport*, which outlines what FGM is, the legislation and penalties involved and the help and support available. This can be downloaded online and is accessible in different languages.

Midwives have a key role to play in safeguarding and providing support to women who have experienced or are at risk of FGM (Raymond, 2015), but as can be seen in the case study, this needs to be done in a sensitive way that does not make assumptions about the woman who has had FGM. FGM is perceived by communities as an 'act of love', undertaken for the betterment of a girl's life and to promote her acceptance into society as a chaste woman, in accordance with cultural precepts. In the immediate aftermath of FGM, a woman or girl may be profoundly shocked by this practice having been arranged by loving parents and a caring community. Women who have undergone FGM have comparable rates of posttraumatic stress disorder (PTSD) as adults who have experienced abuse in early childhood, and 80% suffer from affective or anxiety disorders (WHO, 2018). Psychological complications may include the following:

- psychosexual problems, including sexual dysfunction and low libido
- depression, including possible self-harm and substance misuse
- anxiety
- PTSD

These may be exacerbated or re-awakened during pregnancy, birth and in the postnatal period. Women also need to be aware that any deinfibulation (cutting open the sealed vaginal opening of a woman who has been infibulated, which is often necessary for improving health and wellbeing as well as to allow intercourse or to facilitate childbirth) that takes place during birth cannot be repaired as it is illegal to reinstate any form of FGM. It is vital to consider the possible physical and psychological complications of FGM and how to manage these. If indicated, refer the woman to the obstetric team or mental health services for further assessment.

Sexual abuse

Caring for survivors of sexual abuse can be complex. It may be recent or historical and may be ongoing. For midwives, it is vital to remember that even (what we consider to be) the most innocuous care we give may be triggering for those who have experienced sexual violence or abuse. By its nature, maternity care is intimate and involves physical contact from taking a pulse to internal examinations. Women may choose not to disclose their experiences, but we must still be alert for signs of distress when we are giving care; this may be verbal or non-verbal including body language or avoidance behaviours. As with other issues discussed in this chapter, sexual abuse may be linked to mental ill-health and coping strategies such as self-harm or substance misuse may become apparent. From a midwifery perspective, it is always helpful to reflect on how it must feel to be on the receiving end of care that we consider routine. Regardless of a woman's background and whether she has disclosed trauma of any sort, our words and actions are powerful and we should always be aware of the impact of the care we give.

Definitions

As Table 4.4 demonstrates, sexual violence and abuse includes any behaviour of a sexual nature which is unwanted and takes place without consent or understanding. This includes rape, sexual assault, sexual harassment, childhood sexual abuse, FGM and more.

Table 4.4: **Definitions of sexual violence**

Rape	A rape is when a person uses their penis without consent to penetrate the vagina, mouth or anus of another person. Legally, a person without a penis cannot commit rape, but a female may be guilty of rape if they assist a male perpetrator in an attack.
Assault by penetration	This offence can be committed by either gender and carries the same sentences as rape. Assault by penetration is no less serious than rape.
Sexual assault	This offence can be committed by either gender. Sexual assault is any act of physical, psychological and emotional violation in the form of a sexual act inflicted on someone without their consent. It can involve forcing or manipulating someone to witness or participate in any sexual acts.
	Not all cases of sexual assault involve violence, cause physical injury or leave visible marks. Sexual assault can cause severe distress, emotional harm and injuries that can't be seen – all of which can take a long time to recover from.

The *Sexual Offences Act 2003* (Legislation.gov.uk, 2012) is an act of the Parliament, which came into force on 1 May 2004. It replaced older sexual offences laws with more specific and explicit wording. It also created several new offences such as non-consensual voyeurism, assault by penetration, causing a child to watch a sexual act and penetration of any part of a corpse. It defines and sets legal guidelines for rape in English law. It is also the main legislation dealing with child sexual abuse.

Consent

Sexuality and sexual practices are complex. The key to understanding the issue of sexual abuse and violence is consent; an issue that is often the subject of debate. In a nutshell, without clear consent any sexual act constitutes assault. In order to consent to a sexual act, a person must give permission for it to happen or agree to do something. In addition, the following should be considered:

- Whether they had the capacity to make a choice about whether or not to take part in the sexual activity at the time in question. By capacity, this can mean whether they were old enough, whether they were intoxicated or whether they had the mental capacity to choose (e.g. learning difficulties.)
- Whether they were in a position to make that choice freely, and they were not constrained in any way. This means without physical or mental coercion of any kind (The Survivors Trust, 2020).

The legal age for young people to consent to sex is 16, irrespective of sexual orientation. The aim of the law is to protect the rights and interests of young people and make it easier to prosecute people who pressure or force others into having sex they don't want.

Although the age of consent remains 16, the law is not intended to prosecute mutually agreed teenage sexual activity between two young people of a similar age, unless it involves abuse or exploitation. Young people, including those under 13, will continue to have the right to confidential advice on contraception, condoms, pregnancy and abortion (The Survivors Trust, 2020).

Child sexual abuse

Clearly the issue of consent and the abuse of trust is vital in considering child sex abuse. A child is defined as any person under the age of 18. Child sexual abuse involves forcing or inciting a child to take part in sexual activity, whether or not the child is aware of what is happening and not necessarily involving a high level of violence. This may involve physical contact including rape or oral sex or non-penetrative acts such as masturbation, kissing, rubbing and touching outside of clothing. They may also include non-contact activities, such as involving children in looking at or producing sexual images, watching sexual activities, encouraging children to behave in sexually inappropriate ways, or exploiting or grooming a child in preparation for abuse (including via the internet) or prostitution. Child sexual abuse can be committed by both men and women or other children.

Child sexual exploitation

Child sexual exploitation (CSE) is a form of child sexual abuse. It occurs where an individual or group takes sexual advantage of a child or young person under the age of 18 for his or her own benefit. Power is established through the use of threats, bribes, humiliation or by telling the child or young person that he or she is loved by the perpetrator. A child's or young person's personal, socioeconomic or emotional vulnerability may be used to exploit them. The victim may have been sexually exploited even if the sexual activity appears consensual. CSE does not always involve physical contact; it can also occur through the use of technology. CSE occurs throughout the UK and affects boys as well as girls from any social ethnic or financial backgrounds (NHS England, 2016; The Survivors Trust, 2020).

The impact of sexual abuse and violence

The long-term effects of sexual abuse and violence can include many emotional, psychological and physical conditions, and these may vary from person to person. The experience of sexual assault or abuse at any age irrespective of gender identity can have devastating effects on every aspect of a person's sense of being and life – on the mind, body, behaviour, thoughts and feelings.

A survivor of sexual violence and abuse will often have feelings of guilt, shame, self-blame, embarrassment, fear and distrust of others, sadness or anger, lack of control or denial to name but a few. They will frequently suffer from PTSD, an anxiety disorder caused by very stressful, frightening or distressing events. Someone with PTSD often relives the traumatic event through nightmares and flashbacks and may experience feelings of isolation, irritability and guilt (see Chapter 1 for further information). Other common responses will also include substance misuse, self-harming behaviour, psychotic episodes, borderline personality disorder and relationship problems (The Survivors Trust, 2020).

Case Study 4.3

Jo, a 33-year-old primiparous woman, attends her initial booking appointment at a children centre at 8 weeks' gestation. She attends on her own and appears to be quiet and withdrawn. When you take details regarding her social history, Jo discloses that she was raped at university when she was 18. She reports that she did not report this at the time as she was concerned about the response. Since leaving university, she has had no further contact with the perpetrator. She reports being in a loving, supportive relationship currently; her husband is aware of what happened but finds it difficult to discuss, and it can cause problems within their relationship.

Managing the case study

All types of sexual violence are serious. The law uses different terms such as rape, assault by penetration and sexual assault to differentiate between the types of offence. However, any kind of sexual violence should be taken seriously. Reassure Jo that no matter what has happened to her, the circumstances that it happened in or how long ago the assault occurred, was not her fault. Blame is always with the perpetrator and never with the victim.

It can be hard to hear someone disclose sexual abuse or violence. As midwives we need to remember that our initial response can be crucial in setting the tone and engendering a relationship of trust. A supportive reaction reduces any shame or blame the survivor may feel following the abuse. Encouraging words and phrases can avoid judgement and show support for the survivor. We can acknowledge that the experience must have been traumatic, and we can use phrases such as 'I'm sorry this happened','that must have been very difficult for you' or 'thank you for sharing this with me' to help convey empathy and validate their experience.

As with any complex situation, women will have individual responses to pregnancy and experiences of being pregnant, and as midwives we need to be aware of both the variety of emotions women may experience and the fact that these may change through pregnancy and birth. For some women the experience of pregnancy may not be what they expect; they may be concerned about becoming 'public property', pregnancy itself can trigger a feeling that the baby is 'taking over' the woman's body and there is no escape or she may be afraid of contact with people such as midwives and doctors. The experience of intimate conversations and procedures may cause significant mental and emotional trauma. Other women may enjoy and celebrate pregnancy as a way of reclaiming their bodies and their lives. For many women, there may be a mixture of feelings and emotions all at once or dependent on the stage of the pregnancy or the experience of labour. Regardless of how the woman may be feeling, there are elements of care that can support her in her journey through pregnancy. These include active listening, empathy and awareness of non-verbal signs of trauma or distress. Continuity of the caregiver can be a vital part of building a trusting relationship where the woman does not need to keep repeating her story and potentially reliving her trauma.

It is important to remember that as frontline midwives we are not alone in providing care and support for survivors of sexual violence and abuse. It is good practice to discuss with a survivor whether she feels that a referral to psychological services such as Improving Access to Psychological Therapies (IAPT) or the specialist perinatal mental health service would be beneficial. It is also important to reassure her that no matter what the circumstances, how long ago it happened or who was involved, if at any point she wanted to report what had happened to the police, there are people ready and waiting to listen to her and that she will be believed. Pregnancy can be a time of huge personal change and reassessment. Our role as midwives is to walk alongside women, without pressuring them to any particular course of action.

Modern slavery

Modern slavery is a relatively new term, which includes human trafficking, but also includes other human rights issues such as crimes of slavery, servitude and forced and compulsory labour. This definition is provided in the UK's *Modern Slavery Act 2015* (UK Government, 2015), which introduced the umbrella term (STOP THE TRAFFIK, 2017). Where people are exploited, whether or not they have been recruited or transported for a specific purpose, they could be victims of modern slavery.

Human trafficking and modern slavery are happening every day across the UK, affecting thousands of men, women and children. Victims often require health care services to treat problems such as broken bones caused by accidents on dangerous work sites or sexual health conditions and pregnancy, which may be linked to sexual exploitation. This gives the NHS a unique opportunity to make a difference to these victims' lives (STOP THE TRAFFIK, 2017). For midwives, as with all complex situations, it can be anxiety-provoking to be faced with such situations. We may fear mistakenly identifying issues or missing them completely. We may feel out of our depth when trying to support women in potentially dangerous circumstances. Their lives may be complex, involving sexual violence or abuse as well as exploitation and potentially resulting in substance misuse or mental ill-health. As always, we need to be as well informed as we can be and to understand our local processes of support and referral. Beyond that, however, it is essential that we continue to act within the core tenets of midwifery practice, with safety, care, communication and respect at the heart of what we do.

Useful resources

A free e-learning module has been developed by Health Education England to train NHS staff. This online resource provides an overview of the issue of modern slavery. It is aimed at helping all health care staff recognise the signs that someone has been trafficked and to take appropriate action with confidence.

Case Study 4.4

A woman is brought by ambulance into the Maternity Triage Department on her own. She does not speak any English, so an interpreter is arranged. Through the interpreter, she reports that this pregnancy is unbooked, she has not received any antenatal care to date and she is not sure of her gestation (she is visibly heavily pregnant). When asked she reports that she was aware of the pregnancy but did not access maternity care as she had been travelling for a long time and only arrived in the country 2 days ago. She reports that she is originally from Eritrea, where her parents were killed and she was forced into marriage at the age of 14 years old (13 years ago). She has since fled this situation and made her journey to the UK through different countries, using different methods of transport including plane, train and lorry. She reports having suffered emotional, sexual and physical abuse throughout her journey. She arrived into the UK with no money and has no identification documents. She reports that she does not know where she is and is scared of the people who brought her here.

Managing the case study

First of all, a thorough health assessment of the mother and her unborn baby would need to take place. As English is not the woman's first language, it is important that an interpreter is organised. In this case the woman attended on her own; however, in a similar situation where human trafficking is suspected, it is important that anyone accompanying the woman is not used to translate and is asked to leave so that the woman can be spoken to on her own.

The woman reports that she is concerned for her safety; it is worth exploring this with her further by asking of whom she is scared and what she is scared they may do. Reassure her that she is safe whilst she is in the hospital and that she will not be discharged without a safety plan in place.

Local safeguarding policies and procedures should be followed in this situation, and if you are unsure what to do, speak to your line manager, the maternity co-ordinator and/or a member of the safeguarding team who will be able to support you.

An urgent children's services referral should be made to the local authority where the woman has been residing. Consent should be obtained; however due to the level of risk associated, it is not mandatory in this scenario. Due to the concerns about the woman's safety and her vulnerability, an adult safeguarding referral should also be considered with the woman's consent. Reassure her that these referrals are to safeguard her and her unborn baby and to ensure that she has the appropriate support in place.

Ask the woman if she would like to report what has happened to her to the police. If she does, this can be sensitively arranged whilst she is in the hospital. If she does not, then her wishes should be respected and she should be reassured that at if at any point she changes her mind, this can be facilitated.

The National Referral Mechanism (NRM) is a single framework centred on a multi-agency approach to identify victims of human trafficking and modern slavery and refer them to appropriate support. First responders (including police, immigration authorities, local authorities and certain non-government organisations) can refer all suspected victims to the single competent authority for a decision to be made on whether the individual is a victim entitled to access available support. Health professionals are non-first responders and their duty is to safeguard the woman and make appropriate referrals to first responders, in this case social care or the police. For adults, the NRM is a voluntary process requiring their consent. Even if an individual chooses not to enter the NRM, they may still be a victim of modern slavery or trafficking. For children and young people under 18, consent to go through the NRM process is not required (Crown Prosecution Service (CPS), 2019)

In addition to concerns for the woman's physical health, the trauma that she has endured will also have an impact on her mental health and emotional wellbeing. Symptoms may include PTSD, depression, suicidal ideation, guilt and shame, low self-esteem and confidence, emotional withdrawal and erratic mood changes. Referral should be made to psychological services that can best support her, including, for example, the specialist perinatal mental health team.

The woman should not be discharged from the hospital until a thorough assessment has taken place ensuring her safety and she has appropriate follow-up care arranged.

Substance misuse

As health care practitioners, substance misuse is one area of complex psychosocial care that we may encounter most frequently. Substance misuse can affect women from all walks of life and may involve one or a variety of substances. Different drugs can have different impacts both on the mental and physical state of the person taking them, as well as varying effects on the foetus. It is important to assess each situation on its merits, being aware of potential safeguarding issues and noting that it is not only women with 'chaotic' lives who may need intense support. The judgement of a chaotic lifestyle is a subjective one and stereotyping may affect the care we give and the extent to which we can support women. We may under-estimate the abilities of women whose lives appear very complex and over-estimate the abilities of women who appear to be coping. It is also important to remember that, as we have seen throughout this chapter, women may present with a multiplicity of issues; substance misuse may be cause and effect of mental distress, which may in itself be the result of sexual or domestic abuse, trafficking or other complex factors.

Case Study 4.5

You have been asked to review Toni (who is previously known to your service) who was brought into A+E in the night as she was found sleeping in a public area and thought to be under the influence of illicit drugs. Toni is gravida 8 P6, and all children have been removed from her care. Toni is believed to be still using heroin and other illicit street drugs. A bedside scan has revealed she is approximately 32 weeks' gestation and she has not accessed antenatal care so far in this pregnancy, and as a result she is currently unbooked. The woman has a history of offending behaviour and was in prison at the beginning of her pregnancy.

Managing the case study

Local policies and guidelines should be followed, and your line manager, co-ordinator or member of the safeguarding team should be contacted if you feel you need any advice or support.

Once Toni's initial medical needs have been met for her presentation to the hospital, an initial booking appointment needs to be arranged. Her circumstances should be discussed, including:

- her physical and mental health and her personal, social, educational or employment circumstances (which may trigger a more in-depth assessment) and

* her drug use (including the type used, administration and how often) (NICE, 2017).

If it is thought that Toni is injecting drugs intravenously, screening for hepatitis C should be offered in addition to the routine booking bloods.

Ask Toni if she is receiving support for her substance misuse. If she is not already in receipt of support and would like support, she can be referred to her general practitioner (GP) who can discuss this in further detail with her and arrange treatment. The other option would be to sign-post the woman to her local drug treatment service. In addition to the NHS, there are charities and private drug and alcohol treatment organisations that can help. Following an initial assessment, treatment options will be discussed and a treatment plan agreed with the woman. She will also be signposted to local support groups for her and her family and allocated a key worker who will support her throughout her treatment. Psychological support may also be offered (NHS Choices, 2019).

Top tip

If the woman is having trouble finding appropriate support; FRANK, the drug helpline, can be contacted on 0300 123 6600 to discuss options with her.

Drugs and alcohol can affect a person's mental health, so it is pertinent that this is discussed with Toni and referral(s) to appropriate support services such as talking therapies, women's health counselling, the specialist perinatal mental health service or psychological support through drugs services are made with the woman's consent. This may also uncover the extent to which her history is the result of other issues such as childhood sexual abuse or trauma. This in turn will allow holistic care plans to be developed.

In a scenario such as Toni's there is inevitability multi-agency involvement, with a variety of professionals involved from courts and social workers to the police, health visitors and GP services. As midwives we need to bear in mind our core role of providing care for the pregnant and child-bearing woman, and to ensure that our care remains non-judgemental and supportive. This in itself can be very challenging and requires both self-awareness and a mechanism to support us in debriefing and reflection.

Practice learning point

The following are some of the practical areas of midwifery input appropriate to this scenario:

* *Consider offering routine urine toxicology (with consent) at booking and at follow-up antenatal appointments.*
* *An urgent referral to Children's Services should be made, and Toni should be informed that this is being done and the reason why.*

- *Toni should be referred to the consultant obstetrician and for regular growth scans. Follow-up antenatal care with the midwife should also be arranged. Where possible, continuity of caregiver should be facilitated as this reduces the need for the woman to keep repeating her story and evidence shows that better outcomes for the woman and her baby are achieved (NHS England, 2018). If possible, make antenatal appointments to coincide with consultant appointments and scans to reduce the total number of appointments.*
- *Prior to discharge, Toni should be screened to see if she has accommodation and feels safe to return and only discharged upon confirmation of this.*
- *Toni's GP should be contacted to ensure that he or she is aware of the pregnancy and presentation to the hospital and to see if there is any information that is pertinent to her maternity care.*
- *If it is expected that the baby is likely to need observations for withdrawal or additional support at/following birth, it is good practice to inform the neonatal team in advance so they are aware of the history and can plan care in advance. This can also be discussed with the mother so that she is aware of what to expect following birth and if her baby is not able to stay with her.*

In this scenario, due to the late gestation and potential for the woman to give birth early, multi-disciplinary and multi-agency working is key for effective care and safety planning, ensuring best outcomes for the mother and baby.

Conclusion

This chapter has given key ideas around caring for women with complex social needs, which may be linked to mental health issues. Alongside the specifics of the issues discussed, midwives are reminded of the need for honest, open communication; for treating everyone as a valuable individual; and for working alongside the multi-disciplinary team. Although we may sometimes feel powerless in the face of complexity, by foregrounding the core role of the midwife and adhering to the principles of the *Nursing and Midwifery Council (NMC) Code*, we are able to provide respectful care and support. It is important to remember that however much we may feel we want to solve everything, midwives can only influence situations and provide care within our area of expertise and scope of practice. Our skills of listening, caring and coming alongside individuals are invaluable regardless of the situation. This chapter supports these core skills by giving midwives a range of approaches and resources for their practice tool kit.

POINTS FOR REFLECTION

- *Can you think of a time when you have cared for a woman with complex social issues? If so, what were the effects on her mental health?*
- *Can you identify what factors led the woman to experience social complexity? Was it mental health, life circumstance or a history of abuse?*
- *How did caring for a woman with complex social issues make you feel? What aspect of care provision did you find most challenging?*

References

Crown Prosecution Service. (2019). *Rape and sexual offences. Chapter 2: Sexual offences Act 2003 – principal offences, and sexual offences act* [online]. https://www.cps.gov.uk/crime-info/sexual-offences

Department of Health. (2016). *Female genital mutilation risk and safeguarding – guidance for professionals* [online]. https://assets.publishing.service.gov.uk/government/uploads/system/uploads/attachment_data/file/525390/FGM_safeguarding_report_A.pdf

HM Govt. (2013). *Circular 003/2013: New government domestic violence and abuse definition.* https://www.gov.uk/government/publications/new-government-domestic-violence-and-abuse-definition/circular-0032013-new-government-domestic-violence-and-abuse-definition

HM Govt. (2021). *Statement opposing female genital mutilation.* https://www.gov.uk/government/publications/statement-opposing-female-genital-mutilation

Legislation.gov.uk. (2012). *Sexual offences Act 2003* [online]. https://www.legislation.gov.uk/ukpga/2003/42/contents

National Institute of Clinical Excellence (NICE). (2017). *Recommendations. Drug misuse prevention: Targeted interventions* [online]. https://www.nice.org.uk/guidance/ng64/chapter/Recommendations

National Institute of Clinical Excellence (NICE). (2020). *Domestic violence and abuse – NICE pathways* [online]. http://pathways.nice.org.uk/pathways/domestic-violence-and-abuse

NHS Choices. (2019). *Healthy body* [online]. NHS. https://www.nhs.uk/live-well/healthy-body/drug-addiction-getting-help/

NHS England. (2016). *Child sexual exploitation: Advice for healthcare staff.* NHS England.

NHS England. (2018). *The importance of continuity of carer in maternity services* [online]. https://www.england.nhs.uk/blog/the-importance-of-continuity-of-carer-in-maternity-services/

NSPCC. (2020). *Domestic abuse: Learning from case reviews* [online]. NSPCC Learning. https://learning.nspcc.org.uk/research-resources/learning-from-case-reviews/domestic-abuse.

Raymond. S. (2015). *Female genital mutilation: A handbook for professionals working in health, education, social care and the police.* Shoreham-by-Sea: Pavillion Publishing.

RCM. (2018). Safe places? Workplace support for those experiencing domestic abuse. www.rcm.org.uk

Royal College of Midwives (RCM). (2013). Specialist mental health midwives: What they do and why they matter. https://www.rcm.org.uk/media/2370/specialist-mental-health-midwives-what-they-do-and-why-they-matter.pdf

STOP THE TRAFFIK. (2017). *People shouldn't be bought and sold* [online]. https://www.stopthetraffik.org

The Survivors Trust. (2020). *Pregnancy, birth and parenthood after child sexual abuse – online resource* [online]. https://rise.articulate.com/share/8Oo2-UG-d5Jc5AyjV6rs5iyc4cf5tF88S#/lessons/J9cdkT1gIynqNXHIyhZQoShD-8sOhweeL

UK Government. (2015). *Modern slavery act 2015* [online]. https://www.legislation.gov.uk/ukpga/2015/30/contents/enacted

Webb, C., Pio, M., Hughes, S., Jones, E., Dzhumerska, V., Lesniewska, M.... & O'Leary, R. (2020). *Pathfinder toolkit June 2020* [online]. https://communications.safelivesresearch.org.uk/Pathfinder%20Toolkit_Final.pdf.

Women's Aid. (2019). *The survivor's handbook [online].* Women's Aid. https://www.womensaid.org.uk/the-survivors-handbook/.

World Health Organization. (2018). *Female genital mutilation* [online]. https://www.who.int/news-room/fact-sheets/detail/female-genital-mutilation

Useful contacts

24-hour National Domestic Abuse Helpline 0808 2000 247

LGBT+ Domestic abuse helpline 0800 999 5428

help@galop.org.uk

https://www.womensaid.org.uk/covid-19-coronavirus-safety-advice-for-survivors/

https://www.womensaid.org.uk/information-support/useful-links/

The Survivors Trust offers Pregnancy, Birth and Parenthood after Childhood Sexual Abuse, which is resource to help women who have experienced childhood sexual abuse to prepare for pregnancy, birth and parenthood. This can be found at the following source:

CHAPTER 5

Mental health and cultural perspectives

Cathy Ashwin

Motherhood has been portrayed throughout history as the ultimate fulfilment in life for women, and so for a woman to indicate that this may not be true for her may cause great emotional turmoil. This is particularly relevant when deeply ingrained cultural factors have a strong impact on families and society. However, the ideology of motherhood is not always a 'happily ever after story'. Perinatal mental health spans a wide range of emotions from elation through varying degrees of mood change, anxiety and depression, with severe mental illness manifesting as puerperal psychosis at the far end of the spectrum. Raynor (2014) suggests the transition to becoming a mother can be a time of great vulnerability as it changes the physical and psychosocial aspects of a person. This in turn has an impact on the wider family. These variations in maternal mental health have been discussed in greater depth within other chapters of this book.

This chapter aims to explore mental health and cultural perspectives and how they can be intertwined during the perinatal period. Stigma surrounding mental illness is present in almost all communities, but for some women who live within specific cultural groups there is a very real risk of being ostracised if 'labelled' with a mental illness. These women and their families may become extremely isolated and not seek the help they need for fear of prejudice and stigma associated with mental health. The reasons for this will be explored and cultural differences will be highlighted to offer an intriguing insight into how the construction of societal belief systems within a cultural group can have a negative impact on the woman and her family.

A case study will be included within this chapter to illustrate not only differences but also similarities between cultures that may affect the wellbeing of women during the perinatal period. This woman's voice illustrates how the deeply entrenched fear to 'conform' to the ideals of motherhood can affect not only the woman's wellbeing but also the family around her. Furthermore, these ideals are not restricted to one group of women but translate across class and culture. Names have been changed to protect identity and confidentiality (NMC, 2018).

The role of the midwife

Cultural beliefs are deeply entrenched in the lives of families and communities who are often living within a hierarchical community within their native countries. Midwives are not exempt from the effects of these beliefs. Therefore midwives working within such environments may experience conflicting personal thoughts when supporting women and families during the childbirth continuum. On one hand, the midwife must remain professional and provide sound evidenced-based care; whereas, conversely, she* may struggle with her own deep traditional cultural beliefs potentially giving rise to internal conflict in her working life.

Midwives also work with women and families from different cultures to their own and who have migrated to countries with diverse beliefs and ideals around childbirth. This also sets a challenge for midwives, as they may not be aware of certain traditions and cultural beliefs, steeped in history, that have travelled within the migrant family to a new country and environment. Midwives must be sensitive to these issues and also, importantly, not impose their cultural beliefs upon the woman, which may cause distress through lack of understanding on both sides.

Nonetheless, cultural differences aside, many of the mental health issues and concerns for women in the perinatal period cross all barriers, cultures, classes, ethnicities and parities; as midwives we should be able to give compassionate care to the women and families we encounter. It is also beholden to us as midwives to pursue continuous professional development in order to increase our knowledge and understanding of perinatal mental health (PMH), incorporating cultural diversity. The *UK Nursing and Midwifery Council (NMC) Code*, which governs the professional standards that midwives must uphold to be accountable and registered practitioners, are based around four themes (NMC, 2018).

These themes provide an excellent framework when planning care and must be considered and adhered to in all aspects of women's care, including PMH:

- Prioritise people.
- Practise effectively.
- Preserve safety.
- Promote professionalism and trust.

---

*'She' has been used throughout the chapter for ease; however, we acknowledge this could affect male midwives and caregivers.

The transition to motherhood can be the catalyst for women to experience feelings of overwhelming joy but sometimes unhappiness and sadness or feelings of inadequacy as their independence feels threatened and their position in the family and society has shifted. Midwives can play a key role in supporting the transition by listening to women, building up a relationship so that the woman feels confident in expressing her concerns. To enable this relationship, midwives need to explore their own feelings and cultural beliefs to gain some understanding of the woman's dichotomy of being a good mother and partner and, importantly, being confident in her new perceived position in society.

Professional awareness

Cultural beliefs also extend to caregivers, so midwives may be reluctant to broach the subject of PMH, as this may be alien to their way of life. However, where perceived barriers have been broken down and midwives do wish to ask women about perinatal health, many lack the confidence to support women. Phoosuwan, Lundberg, Phuthomdee, and Eriksson (2020) found that public health professionals (PHPs) felt unable to detect and manage the symptoms of perinatal depression, as they lacked sufficient self-efficacy to provide the support required. These findings emerged from their study which involved training to improve levels of self-efficacy amongst PHPs. The focus groups illustrated the lack of knowledge around PMH concerns as in the following quotes:

> Before SIP (training), I focused only on the pregnant woman's physical health, not on their mental health. But after the intervention programme, I provide more mental health promotion for women (FGD1).

> If we knew the woman was at risk during pregnancy or after childbirth, we would plan with the multidisciplinary team to follow up and provide more specific support to her (FGD3) (Phoosuwan et al., 2020).

The second quote clearly demonstrates a lack of awareness of the issues. Hopefully, if more training such as this can be implemented in other countries, then women across the world may feel more able to disclose their feelings of distress and depression.

This study demonstrated that many health professionals including midwives (although perceiving themselves as caring health providers) did not have an awareness of the issues around PMH. Many of those who did have some perception, however, lacked the courage and confidence to provide or signpost support for the women.

A historical perspective

Historically, cultural traditions have often been associated with religious rituals when transitioning through significant changes in life, with the three most recognised being birth, marriage and, ultimately, death. Rituals help to give meaning and are thought to guide and support families moving from one stage in life to another. In most countries throughout history, the time around childbirth is seen as a potentially dangerous period for a woman and subsequently the child. Therefore many of the cultural beliefs were centred around protecting the woman, thus ensuring her health and safety and that of the baby.

Almost universally, the postpartum period was classed as the 40 days after birth, and we still conform to this today. For many cultures, the woman was made to rest for the 40 days, as in the Muslim community and others. In Islam, a postpartum woman was considered 'unclean' therefore unable to participate in any food preparation for herself or the family (Eberhard-Gran, Garthus-Niegal, Garthus Niegal, & Eskild, 2010). Evidence of similar practices have been noted in Mexico and Latin America, where 40 days' rest was stipulated where very little housework was undertaken and special diets were given to regain health and strength. Eberhard-Gran et al. (2010) have also noted food and rest to be important components of postpartum recovery, with women often returning to childhood homes in many countries, such as Japan, India, Nigeria, Tanzania and Kenya. In addition, gifts were also given to the woman and baby both before and after the birth, as they are in society today. Gifts given before the birth, were not as frequent in many cultures; however, in today's society, the 'baby shower' is becoming more popular, adding pressure for the woman to be happy and consumed with the prospect of 'perfect motherhood'. Held and Rutherford (2012) examined the depiction of motherhood in the popular press and considered the attention surrounding it, arguing that there is still a reluctance to associate perinatal health concerns around childbirth. Cultures can be viewed as both supportive and restrictive in terms of transitioning to motherhood. Gifts were one way of expressing joy at the idea of bringing new life into a family and providing often much needed items such as food, clothing and on occasion tokens such as charms or amulets to protect the baby.

It would appear that all these customs have evolved with the aim to support and nurture the new mother and baby to ensure the healthy continuation of life; however, Gottlieb (1989) would argue that keeping women isolated from the community in the belief they are unclean and a danger to themselves and others could be construed as female oppression. Furthermore, Gottlieb (1989) considers this notion to be rooted in patriarchal societies, this being one reason the traditions existed. Nonetheless, one must consider the benefits of a time of rest, free from the drudgery of everyday household chores, and the provision of nourishing food in maintaining a state of good mental health. Rest and a healthy diet would have also contributed to establishing successful breastfeeding, which in turn alleviates concern around the health of the baby.

Early history in Nordic countries documents the fears of evil spirits that were believed to be all around in nature, and that women needed to be protected from them during the perinatal period (Eberhard-Gran et al., 2010). Again, women in this period were separated from the community as considered carriers of disease and unclean when menstruating or through childbirth. This itself could have stigmatised women and given rise to feelings of unease during this period, although this has not been documented within the literature. Interestingly, women were usually accompanied at night by other women to help ward off evil spirits that might invade and cause harm. Could the devastating effect of puerperal psychosis have been mistaken for evil spirits entering the woman's body? There is no definitive evidence to support the notion, however, only the requisite for women to have another female companion with her during the night. Hanlon, Whitley, Wondimagegn, Alem, and Prince (2009) explored cultural factors affecting pregnant women or new mothers in Nigeria and documented pregnant women being seen as vulnerable and therefore at risk for supernatural afflictions.

The custom of 'churching' is also steeped in a tradition that has almost disappeared in society today, with baptism/christening ceremonies also in decline. Women attended church after their 40 days of seclusion to be reintegrated into society and to be released from the perceived state of unholiness borne from the belief of being unclean and thus vulnerable to disease (Eberhard-Gran et al., 2010).

Many of the customs and rituals remain in the world to a lesser extent; however, customs in some societies have changed. For example, the 'lying-in' period has reduced from 40 days particularly in the Western world, where the majority of pregnant now women give birth in a hospital setting. Some women return home within hours of giving birth and resume normal household activities, depriving them of essential time for rest and recuperation, establishing breastfeeding and eating regular and healthy meals. In addition, women often do not have the benefit of families living close by to provide the additional care to aid physical and mental recovery postpartum. The role of the midwife has been of great value in supporting women through this transition to motherhood and in detecting any mental health concerns early. Sadly, today, the midwife does not always have the capacity to give this care in the community, and lack of close family support may be detrimental in maintaining good mental health. Historical evidence (Cox, 1988) shows that postnatal depression is more likely to occur where postpartum rituals had not been observed. However, we have little evidence to demonstrate whether the observance of strict cultural rituals and enforced seclusion positively impacts PMH or, conversely, whether those rituals adversely affect a woman's mental health. Rest and a healthy diet have been shown to be beneficial in restoring health postpartum; however, to be apart from family, friends and social interaction at such a momentous time may outweigh the good intentions.

Cultural beliefs

For as long as history has been retold, childbirth has been steeped in cultural beliefs and traditions, with many failing to recognise PMH issues. As mentioned previously, childbirth is usually celebrated as a wondrous and joyful event in a woman's life (page 102). However, the role of the woman as a mother can be a source of conflict for some women and not always embraced fully for fear of losing one's identity and position in the workplace. Religious beliefs also have a part to play in suppressing women's anxieties and PMH.

Spanish-speaking people and those from Latin American countries (Latinas) use the term *Marianismo* to describe the 'traditional' female role. Lara-Cinisomo, Wood, and Fujimoto (2019) expand upon this role to include virtue, passivity and putting others first and found that although this did not appear to have an impact on women's mental health during pregnancy, it did contribute to depression in the postnatal period. Religion was often viewed as a protective factor in many cultures; however, it could be contested that the social support within religious communities may be a contributing factor in reducing the incidence of postnatal depression (PND) for these women (Mann, McKeown, Bacon, Vesselinov, & Bush, 2007).

Considering the concept of *Marianismo* for a woman living in today's society can be a cause for great internal turmoil. Historically, when women were expected to remain in the home and become housewives, produce babies and attend to a husband, being subservient and putting others' needs before their own was considered the norm. Women would very rarely step outside of such expectations, so their feelings and emotions were repressed in many situations and any mental health concerns were usually concealed. Women suffering with compromised mental health issues that were too severe to remain behind closed doors were often incarcerated within psychiatric institutions, which were totally unsuitable for women and usually resulted in separation from their babies. Indeed, many women remained in such institutions for many years and in severe cases for life. Therefore to express feelings of anxiety or depression was a serious admission, so many women were unable to talk to anyone for fear of hospitalisation and loss of their babies. In today's society where women are perceived to 'have it all', similarities still exist where PMH concerns are present. Women are now expected to have a career, earn money and contribute to financial demands of lifestyle, whether the lifestyle is affluent or just keeping a roof over their heads and enough food to survive. This position is put into jeopardy when a baby is born, whether the person is financially secure or just existing, the same dilemmas present themselves. In some circumstances, the women who appear externally as confident, capable people can be greatly affected, not wanting to admit to struggling to cope.

Cultural issues all have one thing in common – life changes for a woman once her pregnancy is confirmed and later when the baby is born. Cultural expectations can cause conflict within families, within society and within the workplace. The woman may wish to stay at home and perform the 'traditional' role of a mother and homemaker; however, financial constraints may preclude this desire or she may be afraid of losing her foot on the career ladder of 'success'. On the other hand, if the woman does stay at home, she may feel guilt for not financially contributing and fear being perceived as lazy or work-shy. Staying at home with a baby may not be all the woman thought it would be, and she would rather be at work, finding 24-hour mothering claustrophobic and not intellectually stimulating, but her 'culture' expects the woman to stay at home and not re-enter the workplace.

Religious cultural beliefs also have a part to play in the perception of PMH; for example, in the Israeli Jewish community, there is a strong propensity to hide any sign of mental ill health and avoid seeking medical help. Bina (2014) states generally for this group of women, help is not sought and any feelings of postpartum depression are repressed and couched in a normalisation of the symptoms. Again, the fear of stigmatisation is raised and a fear of judgement precipitating further anxiety in being viewed as an 'unfit' mother. Rather than seek help from a health professional, people suffering with depression lean towards the support of the rabbi or family. Furthermore, Bina (2014) suggests this attitude extends to postnatally depressed women, denying them expert support. Information and studies on this issue are few in Israel; however, reports of PMH concerns are not high, and this raises the question as to whether this is because women gain support from the religious communities or that PMH is an under-reported problem. If the latter, then more needs to be done to encourage women to seek specialised help and break down the cultural barriers preventing such situations because, if untreated, the consequence of poor PMH can have far-reaching negative effects on the future for the woman and her family.

Studies undertaken in urban areas of India and Pakistan (McCauley et al., 2020) demonstrated that women are becoming more enlightened about PMH, but many are still encompassed within cultural beliefs and stigma. They are not forthcoming with health care professionals for fear of repercussion from husbands and family. Gender issues around producing male infants is still a concern and fear for many women, as witnessed by the authors when working in India. Furthermore, McCauley et al. (2020) agree that the gender issue causes stress in some women, as found during interviews with the women in the study. The women were subject to abuse from the family for giving birth to a female infant.

In Japan, help and support are starting to have an impact on the PMH of women, but more work remains to be undertaken to improve the situation. For some Japanese women, the need to repress feelings of anxiety and depression perinatally stems from the fear of being seen as an unfit mother. The recent maternal mortality rate, with suicide being cited as the cause, in Japan was 8.7 per 100,000 births, which is higher than some Western countries (Suzuki, 2018). Many instances of PMH issues are now being addressed, and reliance on family and cultural tradition is less prevalent. Traditionally, a Japanese woman would usually be cared for by her mother and temporarily move back in with her parents; this practice is known as *sa to gae ri bunben* ('home to the village to give birth') (Yoshida, Yamashita, Ueda, & Tashiro, 2001). In today's society, this cultural practice is in decline, and the Japanese government is now beginning to recognise the need to provide more support for women. Tumi, a first-time mother who gave birth in the UK, embraces Western culture and comments on the situation in Japan:

It seems more public awareness of postnatal depression has been raised recently but care for mothers after birth only started in 2017.

The government decided more funds for postnatal care for mothers from 2017. Before that point, main focus of postnatal care was baby and not enough support for mothers. Now all mothers can receive two postnatal check-ups (2 weeks after and a month after birth).

I found a shocking news article – the largest cause of death of pregnant women and women gave birth within one year was suicide. Obviously, there was necessity of more support for those women.

In 2018 only 6.16% of men took paternity leave. Long-working hours are common in Japan. I think it's not unusual that mothers don't have much support from their partners. Social pressure is huge (pushchairs on public transportation and breastfeeding in public space are not welcomed, etc). Many women with small babies can be easily isolated in Japan.

One of the reasons Tumi decided to move to the UK was because she felt more able to participate in her care during pregnancy and birth and to make choices around her care. Having a baby in the UK felt more inclusive to her and gave her more independence from tradition and medicalised birth.

Many cultural traditions share similarities in having a postnatal period of up to 40 days, where mothers are encouraged to rest and not undertake their 'usual' household duties, special foods are eaten and the mother stays together with the baby (Lui, Petrini, & Maloni, 2015; Ma & Kong, 2006). Although many cultural traditions may be questionable in respect to safety, for example, giving birth in an outside building such as a mud hut or stable and using unsterilised implements for cutting the umbilical cord, the practice of 'lying in' may be protective for mental health.

Studies from Nepal (Sharma, van Teijlingen, & Simkhada, 2016) demonstrate that the family and villagers including the local Shaman are involved in the perinatal period, supporting and caring for the woman physically and spiritually; however, no mention of how the woman is feeling emotionally is voiced. One could assume the wraparound care given to these women provides a protective factor against PMH illness. However, the lying-in period can also leave women feeling isolated, unable to leave the house, often staying with family with whom she is not comfortable or familiar such as parents-in-law. Wong and Fisher (2009) argue the feelings of isolation can contribute to postnatal depression and lack of professional help at such times may exacerbate and prolong the situation. Women worldwide continue to struggle with the fine balance of childbirth 'fitting in' on the life continuum. In the UK we are presumed to have the resources and support for women to acknowledge how they are feeling and to not be afraid to seek help, but culture and tradition still prevail in some situations. The following case study illustrates the struggle in maintaining sanity and self-belief following pregnancy and working in what we expect to be a caring community.

Case Study 5.1

Marie (pseudonym used to protect identity as per NMC regulations) worked full time as a midwife and was expecting her first child. She applied for a position to work two nights per week on her return from maternity leave. The head of midwifery considered this to be an unreasonable request and would only agree if Marie returned to work after 6 weeks following the birth. This situation caused great anxiety on several levels. Marie's husband was unsupportive and compounded the situation by implying that the couple would be in financial difficulties if Marie did not return to full-time work. The pregnancy had been a surprise, and for her husband, it was difficult to come to terms with the lifestyle changes a new baby would bring. At the other end of the spectrum, Marie's mother was disapproving of Marie returning to work altogether as she still believed that women should stay at home to care for their babies. Marie became very anxious towards the end of the pregnancy, as she did not feel supported by anyone. She did want to return to work as she loved being a midwife but could not imagine how she could leave a baby so soon after giving birth. The only way to keep her job was to agree to the two nights per week and return after 6 weeks. This conflict with work, her husband and her mother marred the rest of the pregnancy and the weeks and months after. Marie felt she had no one to talk to and felt ungrateful for what she did have in life: a home, baby and family. Following the birth, Marie developed postnatal depression but did return to work after 8 weeks (concession to have 2 weeks annual leave was granted). However, the depression remained untreated, and Marie carried on with life on autopilot for many months, afraid to been seen as not coping. Bonding with the baby was difficult as Marie felt she could not get too attached to him, as it would make returning to work more problematic. The depression continued until Marie became pregnant for the second time and found a midwife who was able to provide appropriate support for her. This time she had more support from family and a different midwifery manager and was able to return to work much later than the first time. The depression was not all-consuming on this occasion but remained in the background and Marie had by now developed strategies to cope.

Marie's story when seen in print gives only a snapshot of the life of a woman undergoing a major life transition and still unable to break free from the cultural beliefs and guilt of having to make decisions that go against family traditions and cultures. The blame for becoming pregnant was put upon Marie by her husband, and she felt the anxiety of upsetting her mother by not wanting to be at home full-time with a baby and the threat of not conforming to supposed NHS rules for return-to-work in a different role. It would appear there is still much work to be done to break down cultural barriers and beliefs in order to better support women through the childbearing journey. Midwives must equip themselves with the skills and knowledge around the cultural context of women's lives to enable them to encourage trusting relationships whereby women feel able to express their feelings.

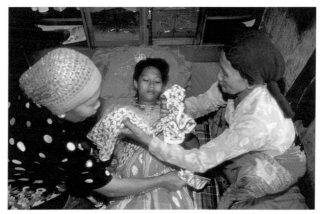

Image 5.1 A young woman prepares for labour and birth accompanied by Traditional Birth Attendants in Nepal. (Courtesy Nancy Durrell-McKenna, Safehands.)

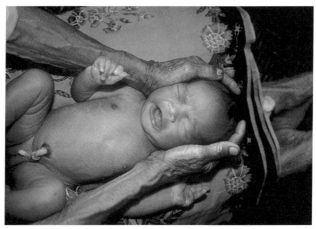

Image 5.2 A newborn infant in Nepal. (Courtesy Nancy Durrell-McKenna, Safehands.)

How cultural beliefs can be a positive influence on wellbeing

The seesaw tips both ways when exploring the benefits or disadvantages of cultural beliefs both through history and in modernity within the experience of childbirth. Midwives must give this consideration when supporting women through the perinatal period and respect the cultural beliefs of the individual women and families. We cannot impose our beliefs or dismiss those of the women, as this could destroy the woman–midwife relationship and risk losing trust and confidence. Ultimately, without openness and honesty, the mental health of the woman in our care could be compromised. As midwives we cannot claim to know the cultural histories of all the women we meet, as we now live and work within such a diverse community.

A prime example of trying to change situations in the belief that it is 'safer' or 'better' for the woman can be seen in Aboriginal communities in the rural and remote areas of Australia. It is very important for Aborigines to stay connected to the land and surrounding flora during pregnancy, birth and beyond. Marriott and Ferguson-Hill (2014) concur that the wellbeing of the woman, baby and her family is firmly rooted in the belief that is connected to their country or homeland. Therefore to birth elsewhere would be detrimental to a woman's mental health. Nonetheless, many women are separated from their families and moved from their usual remote and rural surroundings to give birth in a medical environment many miles away in the belief that this is safer for both mother and baby. To have to move away from the safety net of the family and friends with associated cultural practices is harmful and distressing for the woman. This can have long-lasting negative results for all involved including the mother–child relationship, mental wellbeing and the child's immune system.

Stewart (1999), when discussing cultural practices and childbirth with women of the Warmun community of Western Australia, found a strong belief in the need to protect not only the physical health but also the spiritual health of the woman. Women gave examples through shared stories of birth experiences, explaining that the older women in the camps care for them out of site of the men until they had birthed. They use prayer and warm paperbark to ease the pains of labour. After the birth, the placenta is usually buried. Midwives and allied health professionals must consider these factors when caring for women away from their homeland and try to accommodate their concerns, for example, to enable the woman to take the placenta home to bury or to hold symbolic ceremonies to promote bonding and attachment with the baby. Middleton (2006) states this will enable links to be forged between the homeland, mother and baby. Change is inevitable, and some Aboriginal women will suffer with PMH issues. To support women who may suffer with the changes imposed upon them, Marriott and Ferguson-Hill (2014) advocate appropriate screening tools, such as a the Edinburgh Postnatal Depression Score (EPDS), which has been adapted and utilised with a culturally sensitive approach. Culturally appropriate mental health services should be used for Aboriginal women as initiated by Aboriginal Community Health Services (ACCHS) in Western Australia.

Examples of historical cultural practices have not always been viewed as a positive factor in supporting women during the perinatal period; however, the value of social support and rest cannot be overlooked. LeMasters et al. (2020) explored the practice of *chilla*, the support given to women 40 days postpartum in Pakistan, and found it to be beneficial in protecting against PND. Women who did not participate in *chilla* appeared to be at higher risk of PND and had increased anxiety around role conflict.

Cultural risk factors affecting perinatal mental health

PND can affect any woman during pregnancy, birth and postnatally in varying degrees of distress. Although a cause may not be apparent, many factors have been cited as potential triggers for depression to develop and include poverty, lack of support, partner abuse, unstable relationship and underlying mental health issues. However, these factors can be compounded where there are also cultural factors included. In China, for example, pressure may be placed upon the woman to produce a male baby or the woman may be subjected to unwanted and overbearing intrusion by the partners parents (Li et al., 2020). Furthermore, Li et al. (2020) argue that as the obstetricians in China do not have time to give postpartum health advice, the women rely on cultural tradition. This involves not bathing, eating only hot meals and taking hot drinks and remaining inside the house for 40 days (doing 'the month') (Liu et al., 2015).

A further significant factor that may have contributed to poor PMH was the Chinese law of restricting families to have only one child (Liu et al., 2015). This policy was revoked in 2016, which then allowed two children per household. These policies add extra stress in the desire for a male child. Furthermore, Ma and Kong (2006) argue that because of further cultural practices of increased food intake and lack of exercise during pregnancy to improve the chances of a healthy baby, the rate of caesarean section increased. This in turn, alongside Chinese lifestyle restrictions (i.e. employment concerns), increased the potential for complications post birth and thus increase the risk of PND.

The desire or expectation to produce a male infant is also prevalent in Nigeria, and the risk of PND depression is high in this country. Moreover, Adeponle, Groleau, Kola, Kirmayer, and Gureje (2017) argue that PND is a complex phenomenon exacerbated by cultural practices and social relations.

Being a single parent still holds stigma in Nigeria and to a great extent the fear of repercussions if there is deviation from the traditional customs associated with birth (Hanlon et al., 2009). Although, maternal and child health clinics have midwives working in them, many Nigerian women are still influenced by traditional faith healers within religious settings, Islamic and Yoruba included. Adeponle et al. (2017), in exploring the concept of PMH, asserted that women described their mental health in physical health terms relative to their social circumstances. Examples cited were headaches, childbirth-induced madness, insomnia, stress and blues/depression, and these were attributed to causes such as uncaring partner, in-law problems, wanting a male child, spiritual attack and not resting. A further common link found in the Adeponle et al. (2017) study to emerge is the notion of feeling trapped in the period of confinement, being unable to leave the home, being submissive to care and custom while striving for self-efficacy and control.

Mwape, McGuinness, Dixey, and Johnson (2012) suggest that becoming a mother greatly increases the risk of becoming depressed due to the major adjustment that is made. Their study focused on the lives of women in Zambia and found the incidence of PND greater than in high-income countries and indicated this could be attributed in part to cultural constraints. Perinatal health concerns have not been acknowledged in countries such as Zambia, and thus women have not reported their feelings. Furthermore, Mwape et al. (2012) found similarities in cultural concerns, such as stigma attached to Human immunodeficiency virus (HIV) testing, being forced to live with a partners' family and marital status. Culturally, many, but not all, African men either abandon their pregnant partner or take on more than one wife, compromising the mental health of the woman.

As with many other cultures, Korean women have been cared for by their mother or mother-in-law in the home for up to 3 weeks postpartum; this was known as *Sanhujori* (Song, Chae, Jung, Yang, & Kim, 2020). However, similar to situations in other parts of the world, the nuclear family is not as close today, with families moving away to seek employment and a better way of life. This ultimately has an impact on the wellbeing of women and their families during their childbirth journey. To support women who do not have the benefit of close family, care stand-alone centres have been developed for women and their babies to stay postpartum (Choi & Jung, 2017). These centres, known as *Sanhujoriwan*, are commercial enterprises, and women stay for around 2 weeks following discharge from the hospital. Although on the surface this may seem an ideal opportunity for women to regain their health and establish breastfeeding away from the usual household commitments, the situation is not ideal. Some women take the opportunity to the full extent, which in some cases excludes caring for the baby, and as such, when returning home, the mother is not mentally prepared for caring for a newborn. Partners are permitted to be with the woman in the *Sanhujoriwan* but no other family members. Song and Park (2010) found that women who had used the *Sanhujoriwan* did not cope as well as women who had not used this facility when returning home, reporting higher levels of stress and PND. Further studies are being undertaken to include rooming-in and including the wider family members in the post birth support in the *Sanhujoriwan* to improve long-term outcomes for the family. However, this does not account for the families who are separated from close family members; they may still require additional support.

Barriers to seeking perinatal mental health support

Despite greater exposure of highlighting mental health concerns, many women struggle to acknowledge they are suffering, and midwives are not always made aware of the problem despite the close and unique contact they have with women at this important time (Viveiros & Darling, 2019). Further difficulties in accessing support are evident where midwifery and other health care professionals are not available, and women then rely on family or religious bodies (Bina, 2014). Moreover, Viveiros and Darling (2019) highlight that in some instances, lack of cultural competencies in services (Hauck et al., 2015) and subliminal stigma prevented acceptability of PMH for many (Edge, 2010). The notion of cultural identity can hinder accessing support (Edge, 2010), and seeking help is viewed as something to be ashamed of (Peeler, Stedman, Cheung Chung, & Skirton, 2018).

> **Case Study 5.2 Perinatal mental health in Romanian women living in the UK**
> **Dr Silvia Gerea**
>
> Perinatal mental illness, such as postnatal depression, following childbirth has long carried social stigma in Romania. Women try to hide signs of depression, sometimes with direct consequences, such as when their depressive symptoms turn into thoughts of harming themselves or their babies. In my experience, Eastern-European cultures often place high demand on women to reintegrate quickly into society following childbirth. This may have an impact on mental health as the woman adjusts to the transition of motherhood.
>
> I am of dual citizenship, Romanian and British, and as a psychologist see many Romanian clients who require support with their mental health. Many clients worry that if they involve their general practitioner (GP) or other health professionals with their mental health concerns, they will be reported to social services and their children will be taken away or they

will be investigated by social workers. The majority of Romanian clients feel a fear of the unknown. Not knowing the NHS system or fully understanding care pathways has created many urban stories amongst Romanian communities, such as a fear of being deported to their home country even though they have a legal entitlement to remain in the UK. Therefore it is important to try and alleviate fear and encourage people to make contact with NHS services should they require support for their mental health.

An existing gap was identified around providing perinatal mental health support to women from Romania. This included support for women in the postnatal period who have a place in a *mother and baby unit* and women separated from their babies because of child protection concerns.

Some of the main cultural challenges for Romanian women are a lack of understanding of perinatal mental health and also a lack of joined-up approaches between the NHS perinatal mental health services and cultural specialists.

One way of helping to alleviate fears in the Romanian community is by creating information sessions to explain the actual health care system and allowing them to ask questions about how it works.

This idea was successfully tested a few years ago with input from social workers and professionals all from a Romanian background. We organised free informational seminars in one of the Romanian community centres. This enabled Romanian people to ask questions and also listen to professional presentations. This appeared to improve knowledge and understanding and increase their inclusivity by helping the Romanian community accept the diversity of UK culture.

Romania has a negative tradition of indifference to psychology, psychotherapy and psychiatry, with roots embedded in the communist political system, where mental illness was seen as a disgrace. This type of thinking has been cultivated ever since, and mental illnesses are stigmatized up to this date.

The negative effects of postnatal depression are often exacerbated by a delay in diagnosis and treatment. During my extensive work in the Romanian community in the UK, I have met many women who are reluctant to admit that they feel depressed, fearing that they might be judged as a 'bad mother' or unable to care for their own child. Many do not understand what is happening to them, or that they can access help by talking to their midwife or health visitor.

I explain to the women I see that they need to set aside time to recover from pregnancy and childbirth and adapt to the new role of motherhood. When women give birth to a child, a mother is born too. It is of great importance for health care professionals to understand each

(Continued)

woman's individual context, history and belief systems when treating perinatal mental health problems.

Empowering mothers is important for recovery. Perinatal mental health conditions are illnesses and are not a reflection of the woman as a mother. I always say to my clients, *'You are you and not your illness'.*

Midwives' lack of cross-cultural knowledge within the scope of PMH can be a barrier to supporting women. Viveiros and Darling (2019) expand upon these concerns, suggesting they are exacerbated through language barriers, and that screening tools such as EPDS may not be the panacea for detection of PMH concerns. Women most greatly affected by language barriers are often the most disadvantaged members of society including refugees and ethnic minorities.

McCauley et al. (2020), in exploring the views of women in India and Pakistan, noted that mental health was personal and such information should not be disclosed to health care providers, as this was something to be ashamed of and would make them feel afraid or uncomfortable. However, a few feared that disclosure of mental health concerns would anger their husbands and access to further care would be prevented. Some women felt they could not burden the health care professional with their concerns, as they were already overworked and so could not help them anyway. A further concern was that the women in the study suggested that they would prefer health care professionals to show more empathy towards them and ensure confidentiality was upheld.

Lack of trust in professionals is also a concern which moves both ways where continuity is an issue. Women are afraid of disclosing concerns to someone they have not built up a relationship with, and conversely, midwives can be reluctant to broach the subject for fear of the woman disengaging from help. However, Higgins et al. (2018) argue that midwives should overcome this barrier and to approach women with greater confidence. Competence can be achieved through specialised further training that will equip midwives with the tools to discuss PMH with women.

Connecting themes

All countries have a history of ritual traditions and practices associated with childbirth, and although this chapter has not gone into detail around the rituals performed such as warding off evil spirits with the use of amulets, trinkets and specific ceremonies, it is apparent that some of these practices cross nationalities in varying forms.

Furthermore, many of the same concerns affect women everywhere and contribute to the manifestation of poor PMH, leading to depression, as listed in the following table (Table 5.1).

Table 5.1: **Similarities across cultures with the potential to impact on perinatal mental health**

Situation	Context
Sex of child	Male child preferred (even in some Western cultures)
In-laws/parents	Can be seen as supportive or harmful to mental wellbeing
Marital situation	Stigma if unmarried
Finances	Fear of domestic abuse/violence
Health	Can be supportive
Nutrition	Financial hardship as a burden
Support	Good physical health can be protective but not guaranteed – some cultures advise against exercise at this time
Self-efficacy	Midwifery support not always available
	Protective factor but hard to achieve in oppressive circumstances

Some countries do not have the benefit of fully trained midwives for women during this important period in their lives, and even less have midwives who are specialised in PND and as such do not seek treatment. As noted, women in Nigeria often blame themselves for how they are feeling, and that their life choices are the cause of depression. In countries such as the UK, midwives must be alert to the fact that some women have migrated here and as such be prepared to educate and support them and to signpost to appropriate help if the work is beyond their scope of practice (NMC, 2018).

Summary

Cultural beliefs can impact on a woman's mental health during the perinatal period and may have a positive or negative effect on wellbeing during this time. Through exploring the different ways that women have been cared for through time and culture, similar practices emerge. The need for rest and a good diet would appear to be a universal belief, and rest and a good diet aid the woman's recuperation and the establishment of breastfeeding. However, where this takes place is not always in the best interests of the woman and family and can cause needless stress and anxiety. The role of the partner must be considered; in some cultures, the partner's presence and input are largely ignored, which some would perceive as detrimental to the new family structure. Some of these perspectives and practices are deeply ingrained in the subconscious mind and encapsulate strong emotions belonging to more than the recognised traditions we usually associate within our own cultures. This has been illustrated with the perspectives taken from examples around the world of how childbearing women are considered in various situations. As midwives, we must first examine our own beliefs and cultural practices, which may or may not align with the women and families we care for. We must uphold professionalism and confidentiality and not let our own beliefs impinge on the care we provide. As health care professionals, we must remain impartial, unless the safety of the mother or baby are at risk.

Women must feel able to talk freely without fear or judgement, and it is our duty of care to gain an understanding of different cultural perspectives to enable us to give high-quality midwifery care to all. When utilising tools to assess PMH such as the EPDS, midwives must be mindful of the woman's cultural background and any language barriers hindering a true assessment to be undertaken. Lack of understanding may delay or even prevent appropriate therapy and treatment being offered. Where possible, continuity of care should be given so that an honest and meaningful relationship can develop between the woman and midwife to enable truthful and open discussion to take place. Ultimately, although some women will suffer perinatal mental illness, having insight into cultural issues that may impinge on the health of women will contribute to planning appropriate midwifery care and signposting where greater support is required.

POINTS FOR REFLECTION

- *How could you approach the subject of perinatal mental health with a women from a different culture to where she is living now?*
- *If you are caring for a woman from a different culture to your own, would you feel comfortable asking about her mental health?*
- *Consider how you could validate the woman's feelings to help her disclose her concerns.*
- *Thinking about the midwife's story, consider what alternative options could have been explored to help Marie in this situation.*

References

Adeponle, A., Groleau, D., Kola, L., Kirmayer, L. J., & Gureje, O. (2017). Perinatal depression in Nigeria: Perspectives of women, family caregivers and healthcare providers. *International Journal of Mental Health Systems, 11*, 27. https://doi.org/10.1186/s13033-017-0134-6.

Bina, R. (2014). Seeking help for postpartum depression in the Israeli Jewish Orthodox community: Factors associated with use of professional and informal help. *Women & Health, 54*(5), 455–473. https://doi.org/10.1080/03630242.2014.897675.

Choi, H. K., & Jung, N. O. (2017). Factors influencing health promoting behavior in postpartum women at Sanhujoriwon. *Korean Journal of Women Health Nursing*, 23(2), 135–144.

Cox, J. L. (1988). The life event of childbirth: Sociocultural aspects of postnatal depression. In R. Kumar & I. Brockington (Eds.), *Motherhood and mental illness* (pp. 2). London: John Wright. Causes and Consequences.

Eberhard-Gran, M., Garthus-Niegal, S., Garthus Niegal, K., & Eskild, A. (2010). Postnatal care: A cross-cultural perspective. *Archives of Women's Mental Health*, 13, 459–466. https://doi.org/10.1007/s00737-010-0175-1.

Edge, D. (2010). Falling through the net – Black and ethnic minority women and perinatal mental health care: Health professionals' views. *General Hospital Psychiatry*, 32, 17–25. https://doi.org/10.1016/j.genhosppsych.2009.07.007.

Gottlieb, A. (1989). Rethinking female pollution: The Beng of Côte d'ivoire. *Dialect Anthropology*, 14, 65–79.

Hanlon, C., Whitley, R., Wondimagegn, D., Alem, A., & Prince, M. (2009). Postnatal mental distress in relation to the sociocultural practices of childbirth: An exploratory qualitative study from Ethiopia. *Social Science and Medicine*, 69, 1211–1219.

Hauck, Y., Kelly, G., Dragovic, M., Butt, J., Whittaker, P., & Badcock, J. C. (2015). Australian midwives' knowledge, attitude and perceived learning needs around perinatal mental health. *Midwifery*, 31, 247–253.

Held, L., & Rutherford, A. (2012). Can't a mother sing the blues? Postpartum depression and the construction of motherhood in late 20th-century America. *History of Psychology*, 15(2), 107–123. https://doi.org/10.1037/a0026219.

Higgins, A., Downes, C., Monahan, M., Gill, A., Lamb, S. A., & Carroll, M. (2018). Midwives and nurses addressing mental health issues with women during the perinatal period: The Mind Mothers Study. *Journal of Clinical Nursing*, 27(9–10), 1883–1972. https://doi.org/10.1111/jocn.14252.

Lara-Cinisomo, S., Wood, J., & Fujimoto, E. M. (2019). A systematic review of cultural orientation and perinatal depression in Latina women: Are acculturation. *Marianismo, and religiosity risks or protective factors? Archives of Women's Mental Health*, 22, 557–567.

LeMasters, K., Andrabi, N., Zalla, L., Hagaman, A., Chung, E. O., Gallis, J. A., … Maselko, J. (2020). Maternal depression in rural Pakistan: The protective associations with cultural postpartum practices. *BMC Public Health*, 20, 68. https://doi.org/10.1186/s12889-020-8176-0.

Li, Q., Yang, S., Xie, M., Wu, X., Haung, L., Ruan, W., & Lui, Y. (2020). Impact of some social and clinical factors on the development of postpartum depression in Chinese women. *BMC Pregnancy and Childbirth*, 20, 226. https://doi.org/10.1186/s12884-020-02906-y.

Liu, Y. Q., Petrini, M., & Maloni, J. A. (2015). "Doing the month": Postpartum practices in Chinese women. *Nursing and Health Science*, 17(1), 5–14.

Ma, G., & Kong, L. (2006). *China nutrition and health survey report 2006 Guang-zhou* (pp. 130–218). People's Medical Publishing House Press.

Mann, J. R., McKeown, R. E., Bacon, J., Vesselinov, R., & Bush, F. (2007). Religiosity, spirituality and depressive symptoms in pregnant women. *International Journal of Psychiatry and Medicine, 37*, 310–313.

Marriott, R., & Ferguson-Hill, S. (2014). Perinatal and infant mental health and wellbeing (2nd ed., pp. 337–353). In P. Dudgeon, H. Milroy, & R. Walker (Eds.), *Working together: Aboriginal and Torres Strait Islander mental health and wellbeing principles and practice* (Vol. 19, pp. 337–353)

McCauley, M., Avais, A. R., Agrawal, R., Saleem, S., Zafar, S., & van den Broek, N. (2020). 'Good health means being mentally, socially, emotionally and physically fit': Women's understanding of health and ill health during and after pregnancy in India and Pakistan: A qualitative study. *BMJ Open Access, 10*, e028760. https://doi.org/10.1136/bmjopen-2018-028760.

Middleton, K. J. (2006). Mothers, Boorais and special care: An exploration of Indigenous health workers' perceptions of the obstetric and neonatal needs of rural Victorian Aboriginal and Torres Strait Islander families transferred to the Mercy Hospital for Women (discussion paper No One mda Vic Health Koori Unit) (2nd ed., pp. 337–353). In P. Dudgeon, H. Milroy, & R. Walker (Eds.), *Working together: Aboriginal and Torres Strait Islander mental health and wellbeing principles and practice* (Vol. 19, pp. 337–353)

Mwape, L., McGuinness, T., Dixey, R., & Johnson, S. E. (2012). Socio-cultural factors surrounding mental distress during the perinatal period in Zambia: A qualitative investigation. *International Journal of Mental Health Systems, 6*, 12. http://www.ijmhs.com/content/6/1/12.

Nursing and Midwifery Council (NMC). (2018). *The Code: Professional standards of practice and behaviour for nurse, midwives and nursing associates.* Retrieved May 07, 2020 from https://www.nmc.org.uk/globalassets/sitedocuments/nmc-publications/nmc-code.pdf.

Peeler, S., Stedman, J., Cheung Chung, M., & Skirton, H. (2018). Women's experience of living with postnatal PTSD. *Midwifery, 56*, 70–78. https://doi.org/10.1016/j.midw.2017.09.019.

Phoosuwan, N., Lundberg, P. C., Phuthomdee, S., & Eriksson, L. (2020). Intervention intended to improve public health professionals' self-efficacy in their efforts to detect and manage perinatal depressive symptoms among Thai women: A mixed-methods study. *BMC Health Services Research, 20*, 138. https://doi.org/10.1186/s12913-020-5007-z.

Raynor, M., & Oates, M. R. (2014). Chapter 25: Perinatal mental health. In J. Marshall, & M. Raynor (Eds.), *Myles textbook for midwives* (16th ed., Vol. 25, pp. 531–553). China: Churchill-Livingstone Elsevier.

Sharma, S., van Teijlingen, E., & Simkhada, P. (2016). Dirty and 40 days in the wilderness: Eliciting childbirth and postnatal cultural practices and beliefs in Nepal. *BMC Pregnancy and Childbirth, 16*, 147. https://doi.org/10.1186/s12884-016-0938-4.

Song, J. E., & Park, B. L. (2010). The changing pattern of physical and psychological health, and maternal adjustment between primiparas who used and those who did not use Sanhujory facilities. *Journal of Korean Academy of Nursing, 40*(4), 503–514.

Song, J. E., Chae, H. J., Jung, M. K., Yang, J. I., & Kim, T. (2020). Effects of maternal role adjustment program for first time mothers who use postpartum care centers (*Sanhujoriwon*) in South Korea: a quasi-experimental study. *BMC Pregnancy and Childbirth, 20*, 227. https://doi.org/10.1186/s12884-020-02923-x.

Stewart, M. L. (1999). Ngalangangpum Jarrakpu Purrurn, mother and child: The women of Warmun as told to Margaret Stewart. In P. Dudgeon, H. Milroy, & R. Walker (Eds.), *Working together: Aboriginal and Torres Strait Islander mental health and wellbeing principles and practice* (2nd ed., Vol. 19, pp. 337–353).

Suzuki, S. (2018). Recent status of pregnant women with mental health disorders at a Japanese perinatal center. *The Journal of Maternal-Fetal & Neonatal Medicine, 31*(16), 2131–2135.

Viveiros, C. J., & Darling, E. K. (2019). Perceptions of barriers to accessing perinatal mental health care in midwifery: A scoping review. *Midwifery, 70*, 106–118.

Wong, J., & Fisher, J. (2009). The role of traditional confinement practices in determining postpartum depression in women in Chinese cultures: A systematic review of the English language evidence. *Journal of Affective Disorders, 116*, 161–169.

Yoshida, K., Yamashita, H., Ueda, M., & Tashiro, N. (2001). Postnatal depression in Japanese mothers and the reconsideration of 'Satogaeri bunben'. *Paediatrics International, 43*, 189–193.

Further reading

Queensland Health

Multicultural Clinical Support Resource – Cultural dimensions of pregnancy, birth and post-natal care. https://www.health.qld.gov.au/__data/assets/pdf_file/0035/158669/14mcsr-pregnancy.pdf

West London Mental Health NHS Trust – Cultural competency tool kit. https://www.yumpu.com/en/document/read/49776540/cultural-competency-tool-kit-west-london-mental-health-nhs-trust

Useful information on cultural and community customs, for example, dress, female genital mutilation (FGM) and birth.

NHS Health Education in England. Cultural Competence e-learning modules. https://www.e-lfh.org.uk/programmes/cultural-competence/

Multi-cultural resources

Cox, J., Holden, J., & Henshaw, C. (2014). *Perinatal mental health: The Edinburgh Postnatal Depression Scale (EPDS) manual* (2nd ed.). London: RCP Publications. The second edition of the EPDS manual includes the EPDS questionnaire itself in over 50 other languages, plus a discussion of the questionnaires cultural validity.

Postpartum Support International. (2021). *Perinatal mood & anxiety disorders resources in other languages*. https://www.postpartum.net/resources/resources-in-other-languages/

Translated mental health resources. https://www.beyondblue.org.au/who-does-it-affect/multicultural-people/translated-mental-health-resources

Embrace Multicultural Mental Health (the Embrace Project) is run by Mental Health Australia and provides a national focus on mental health and suicide prevention for people from culturally and linguistically diverse (CALD) backgrounds. They have a range of information in different languages. http://mental.dev-box.com.au/about-us

Multilingual resources for midwives. https://www.mamaacademy.org.uk/for-midwives/multilingual-resources/

Watson, H., Harrop, D., Walton, E., Young, A., & Soltani, H. (2019). A systematic review of ethnic minority women's experiences of perinatal mental health conditions and services in Europe. *PLoS One, vol. 14* https://discover.dc.nihr.ac.uk/content/signal-000762/maternal-mental-health-ethnicity-and-culture

Royal College of Psychiatrists Report. (2015). *CR 197 Perinatal mental health services. Recommendations for the provision of services for childbearing women.* https://www.rcpsych.ac.uk/docs/default-source/improving-care/better-mh-policy/college-reports/college-report-cr197.pdf?sfvrsn=57766e79_2

Special considerations

- Perinatal mental health services will need to serve one or more minority ethnic communities. Such communities may have cultural or religious beliefs and practices that affect marriage and kinship, practices surrounding the birth and early postpartum period and childrearing. These should be respected, provided they are compatible with the wellbeing and safety of the mother and child. It is essential that perinatal mental health clinicians have knowledge and understanding of the cultural beliefs and practices of the communities they serve.
- Asylum seekers and refugees may have experienced trauma and torture and may have lost or been separated from family including their own children. In addition, they may be facing current deprivation and adversity as well as fear of deportation. Their mental health problems may be compounded by grief and posttraumatic stress disorder.

Perinatal mental health services should ensure these patients have access to the additional psychological, social and legal help they require.

• Hanley, J. (2015). *Listening visits in perinatal mental health: A guide for health professionals and support workers*. Routledge. Chapter 7 has some specific guidance on cultural experiences, for example, using a translator phone app or Google Translate to equip you with a range of relevant questions or phrases.

Sources of perinatal mental health training courses

https://www.e-lfh.org.uk/wp-content/uploads/2019/09/Perinatal-Mental-Health-Training-Scoping-Exercise-Nous-Group-Directory.pdf

Edited by: Ranjana Das with Contributions from: Daniel Beszlag, Louise Davies. (2009). Migrant mothers' mental health communication in the perinatal period

http://epubs.surrey.ac.uk/852845/1/Migrant%20Mothers%27%20Perinatal%20Mental%20Health%20Communication.pdf

Some useful insights into real experiences and barriers and a look at use of technology.

Watson, H., & Soltani, H. (2019). Perinatal mental ill health: The experiences of women from ethnic minority groups. *British Journal of Midwifery*, 27(10) https://www.magonlinelibrary.com/doi/abs/10.12968/bjom.2019.27.10.642.

Brookes, H., Coster, D., & Sanger, C. (2015). Baby steps: Supporting parents from minority ethnic backgrounds in the perinatal period. *Journal of Health Visiting*, 3(5) https://www.magonlinelibrary.com/doi/full/10.12968/johv.2015.3.5.280.

Zero to Three. Infant mental health and cultural competence.

https://www.zerotothree.org/resources/1599-infant-mental-health-and-cultural-competence

Example of good practice

Haamla is a unique service that provides essential support for pregnant women and their families from minority ethnic communities, including asylum seekers and refugees, throughout their pregnancy and postnatal period. It aims to improve access within maternity services, empower and inform women of the choices available during their pregnancy and birth, thereby improving health and wellbeing.

https://www.leedsth.nhs.uk/a-z-of-services/leeds-maternity-care/meet-the-team/haamla-service/

CHAPTER 6

Parent–infant relationship

Maureen Doretha Raynor and Helen Griffiths-Haynes

Introduction

In the context of perinatal mental health (PMH), it is of little surprise that the significance of the parent–infant dynamic relationship to child development is well documented. This is because maternal and paternal mental illness such as depression can have a deleterious effect on the emotional wellbeing and psychosocial development of children. It is also possible that the illness has an impact on parenting capacities, which is at the core of this chapter. Midwives, as key public health professionals, have repeated contact with women and their families during the perinatal period, and are well placed to provide effective and compassionate care. An underlying comprehension of the consequences of perinatal mental illness (PMI) and means to promote mental health is a seminal part of the midwife's role and is key to supporting families. Knowledge of how pre-existing or new PMI can disrupt the parent–infant relationship and family dynamics in the early perinatal period, especially as parents transition to their parenting role, will be emphasised.

The chapter aims to do the following:

+ Provide an overview of the parent–infant relationship and why it matters in the context of PMH. This will be done against the background of relevant and influential reports that act as key drivers for change, such as the National Institute for Health and Care Excellence (NICE, 2014) guidelines, *Better Births* (NHS England, 2016a), the National Health Service (NHS) Plan (NHS England, 2019) and the 5-year forward planning report from the Mental Health Task Force (NHS England, 2016b).
+ Explore attachment theories and emerging areas of research.
+ Highlight some notable effects of PMI and trauma on:
    + Child development
    + The parent–infant relationship using a case study to reinforce key points
+ Examine the transition to fatherhood.
+ Discuss the importance of social support as a means of social capital, along with helpful strategies for parents during the perinatal period.

Some key drivers for change

The important and now ubiquitously cited report by NHS England (2016a) *Better Births*, a national maternity review, established a clear vision for maternity services across England. Its emphasis is on a safer, more personalised, kinder, professional, more woman-centred and family-friendly service, where every woman has access to information to empower her to make informed and valid decisions about her care. It focuses on a service that would ensure that a woman, her partner, their baby and immediate family can access support that is centred on their unique individual needs and circumstances.

Since the publication of *Better Births* (NHS England, 2016a), the NHS and its partners have formed an alliance through the national Maternity Transformation Programme to implement its vision for safer and more personalised care across England. This ambitious and targeted programme seeks to achieve the vision set out in *Better Births* by bringing together a wide range of organisations to lead and deliver across 10 work streams. As can be seen from Fig. 6.1, improving access to perinatal mental health

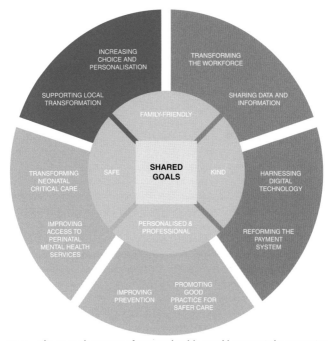

Fig 6.1 The 10 work streams of NHS England (2016a,b) Better Births Maternity Transformation Programme.

(PMH) services features as one of the key work streams. This is a joint initiative between the Maternity Transformation Programme and the Mental Health Programme. At its core is the drive to improve access for women and their families to high-quality specialist PMH care closer to where they live that can provide care and support during the perinatal period.

Vision of the NHS Long Term Plan

The NHS Long Term Plan (NHS England, 2019) identified that approximately one in four women experience a mental health problem during pregnancy and in the first year after giving birth, with anxiety disorders and depression being the most common. The report also raised the spectre regarding the consequences of these women and their families not being able to access specialist PMH service. The chief ambition of these social policies/government reports is to ensure that every family is afforded the opportunity to have the best start in life when a new baby and existing children are factored in the equation.

Transition to parenthood

A new baby brings disruption to the lives of parents, existing children and the wider family unit. Mothers and fathers/partners may find coping with the demands of a new baby both exhilarating and exhausting at the same time. This is because a new addition to the family brings changes, role adjustment and role conflict that might culminate with increased levels of stress and anxiety. The transition to parenthood that accompanies the birth of a first child often results in a real shift in a couple's relationship (Ayers and Sawyer, 2019 and Bouchard, 2014). Social networks are disrupted and so too can be the amount of social support. This may leave some mothers and fathers feeling socially isolated, as caring for a baby leaves very little time for the pursuit of leisure activities. The couple's relationship shifts from a dyad to a triad, becoming more baby-centred. A myriad of issues may result in unhappiness, for example, sleep disturbances, which is inevitable with a new baby. The sleeping pattern of the baby will often act as a barometer for the mood of the parents, especially the mother. A baby's needs have to be met 24/7 with soothing, comforting, feeding, bathing and so forth. Parents may feel sleep deprived with the round the clock demand of caring for a baby. The feeling of loss of self-identity is real, and some parents may grieve for their former life. As day-to-day existence becomes baby-centred, there is a shift in the couple's relation, and fathers/partners might feel pushed out or neglected. Tiredness coupled with sheer exhaustion affect libido and may lead to despair, unhappiness and relationship discord, especially if there were pre-existing financial and relationship difficulties (Rholes & Paetzold, 2019).

This is further compounded if the baby is perceived as a 'crying baby' who is difficult to pacify. Moreover, if the mother is struggling to breast-feed, has had an operative birth, has twins or higher multiples or has experienced pregnancy or labour/birth complications such as antepartum haemorrhage, pre-eclampsia, complex perineal trauma or an unplanned caesarean section, she will need time to recover and become herself again. These issues are important when considering the start of the parent–infant relationship.

The parent–infant relationship: The impact of perinatal mental illness and trauma on infant and child development

The early interaction between parents and their newborn baby is of the utmost importance. Not only does it create a stimulating social learning environment for the infant to thrive, but also it fosters security and positive attachments in the development of the infant. Attachment can simply be defined as a special and lasting emotional connection between an infant and a primary caregiver or nurturer, which serves to promote survival by allowing the infant to feel safe, secure, loved and protected. This resonates with Ainsworth (1979) and Bowlby (1969) definition of attachment of a deep and enduring emotional tie, bond or lasting psychological connectedness that unites human beings across time and space.

The World Health Organization (WHO, 2015) identifies that in the postnatal period, poor maternal mental health is a great source of suffering and in addition may increase the overall risks of morbidity and mortality, as the mother may not be able to feed or care for herself adequately. Neonates are equally likely to be affected, not only physically but also emotionally, as they are so highly sensitive to their environments. Essential bonding activities such as breastfeeding and infant care and interaction, which help mothers and babies to develop a secure and healthy attachment, have the potential to be impacted. This may have consequences for early, later and adolescent development, as well as adult relationships and intergenerational effects.

Basic concepts of attachment theory

Attachment theory is largely based upon the joint work of Mary Ainsworth, an American-Canadian developmental psychologist, and John Bowlby, a British psychologist and psychoanalyst, who collaborated on a body of work spanning the 1950s through to the late 1970s. Although other researchers have since furthered the study of attachment greatly, it is still largely Ainsworth and Bowlby's work which is considered seminal in the field (Gillath, Karantzas, & Fraley, 2016). Drawing initially upon ethnology, cybernetics, control systems, developmental psychology and psychoanalysis, Ainsworth and Bowlby (Bretherton, 1992) created and tested the principles of their theory, which came to radically change thinking about the ways that maternal–infant attachments are formulated and also how they are impacted by separation, trauma, grief and neglect. The fundamental principle of attachment theory arises from Bowlby's initial observations that when babies and children are separated from their mothers, they show signs of distress and anxiety, and that this is not relieved by the presence or attention of other, even very familiar caregivers (Bretherton, 1992). In contrast to other theories of the time, which stated that attachment is a learned behaviour, and that children will respond to whoever feeds them (Dollard & Miller, 1950), Bowlby (1969) theorised that attachment served an evolutionary purpose, and that babies were born pre-programmed to form intense attachments to a primary and singular caregiver, ideally their mothers. Although the possibility of a non-maternal primary attachment figure was not ruled out, Ainsworth and Bowlby (Bretherton, 1992) said that the mother–infant relationship was of key importance because it was not born simply out of a requirement for food, which could be provided by any member of the tribe or community if separation from the mother occurred, but out of a need for responsiveness and emotional connectivity. Additionally, they claimed that the mother–infant dyad was uniquely and specifically programmed to create this bond. This singular maternal attachment figure forms a secure base from which the child explores the world and which supports the formation of healthy and secure social relationships throughout the lifespan. The well-documented research by Ainsworth and Bowlby (Bretherton, 1992) found that disruption of this attachment figure relationship through loss of or by separation from the mother, and the resultant failure to develop a healthy and secure attachment bond, could have severe consequences for the child's emotional and psychological development. They called this phenomenon 'maternal deprivation' and found that it has a particular impact between the ages of 0 and 2 years of age, when the child's brain is undergoing specific stages of development and is linked with the potential for cognitive and emotional impairment, compromised educational development and the inability to form secure adult relationships in later life (Bowlby, 1958). Children who develop healthy and secure relationships with their mothers are generally said to have developed a secure attachment, whilst those who experience disruption to this primary relationship dynamic, and who experience consequences, are said to have developed an insecure attachment (Bowlby et al., 1956). Through a series of experiments, Ainsworth and Bell (1970) observed the responses of children aged 12–18 months of age to a 'strange situation' whereby they were left alone with a stranger by their mothers for a short period of time. It was noted that children who were securely attached coped well with the situation, displayed proximity-seeking behaviours in looking for their mother, avoided the stranger when their mother was not present and happily and quickly re-established connection with her on her return. Conversely, children with an insecure attachment displayed overly distressed or anxious behaviour when the mother left, exaggerated or diminished proximity-seeking behaviours and were angry with the mother on her return or were distrustful and avoided re-connection. These insecure behaviours resulting from an impaired attachment bond with the mother are thought to show the evidence of compromised emotional and neurological development and have the potential to impact the child's ongoing emotional regulation and mental health, cognitive development and future adult romantic and familial relationships (Mikulincer & Shaver, 2012).

Despite critique of the work of Ainsworth and Bowlby in the intervening years, particularly by Schaffer and Emerson (1964) and Rutter (1979) who argued that there were other factors that needed to be considered, more recent research continues to support their work. Marryat and Martin (2010) found that the relationship between healthy attachment and normal child development remained statistically significant even after controlling for socioeconomic factors and family characteristics. Similarly, the WHO (2004) stresses the importance of secure maternal–infant attachment in promoting healthy child development. The Baby Friendly Initiative (UNICEF, 2013, 2019) cites the work of Bowlby (1969) and the subsequent research on attachment theory as evidence and rationale for its standards and as essential knowledge for students, midwives and health care practitioners in implementing them.

Maternal mental health and maternal–infant attachment

Research conducted into the factors that are most likely to affect the development of healthy maternal–infant attachment has shown that poor maternal mental health is significant, and that a healthy emotional climate in childhood is a precursor to the development of a healthy emotional adulthood (Marryat & Martin, 2010). In particular, there is a documented relationship between the early onset and persistence of maternal depressive symptoms such as low mood, social withdrawal, irritability, impaired concentration, hopelessness, guilt, anxiety and childhood maladaptation (Grace & Sansom, 2003). Although it would not be true to say that all cases of maternal depression result in an insecurely attached child, overall maternal depression is considered to be related, with a meta-analysis by Atkinson et al. (2000) finding there to be modest association.

At 18 months of age, the child of a mother experiencing depression in the postpartum period is 5.4 times more likely to display the symptoms of insecure attachment compared with mothers who did not experience symptoms (Grace & Sansom, 2003). Marryat and Martin (2010) found that childhood development was significantly negatively affected by maternal mental health problems, and that there was a direct relationship between the degree of exposure and the severity of symptoms and developmental outcomes for the child. In addition, the early cessation of breastfeeding was more likely. Research by Toth et al. (2009) suggests that some of the behaviour displayed by the mother as a result of the symptoms of depression such as a lack of emotional responsiveness, connection, reassurance and nurturance make it much more difficult for children to develop a secure attachment relationship with their mother, and that maternal depression contributes to children developing negative perceptions of themselves and others. Toth et al. (2009) also found that the quality of the early attachment relationship has a direct effect on the internal concept of the self. In cases of maternal depression where the quality of the relationship was poor, the caregiver was more likely to be perceived by the child as displaying rejecting or abandoning behaviours, and the child was more likely to conceive of themselves as unlovable. Conversely, nurturant parents without depressive symptoms were more likely to raise children who went on to develop positive views of the self and others. Murray et al. (1996) found mothers experiencing depression were less attuned to their baby's needs, were less affirming and were more negating of infant experience. It is unsurprising therefore that in its review, *The Importance of Caregiver-Child Interactions for the Survival and Healthy Development of Young Children*, the WHO (2004) identified that one of the greatest barriers to the natural emergence of a healthy, caring relationship that meets the child's attachment needs is caregiver mood and emotional state.

The effects on child development

With regard to the emotional growth and development of the child, research suggests that depression in the postpartum period has a clear effect in infancy, but more longitudinal effects are less clear. There is no conclusive evidence to suggest exactly how the impact of maternal mental health problems and insecure attachment changes over the child's lifespan, as responses are individual and variable (Marryat & Martin, 2010). Thus more research in terms of longitudinal studies are needed in this area. Yet, there is a growing body of evidence that suggests that the effects of poor maternal mental health and insecure attachment may carry forward into later childhood and, indeed, adulthood. It is probable that the greatest effects are seen in mother–infant dyads experiencing chronic, long-term or recurrent issues. The good news as the literature suggests is that effective treatment and support may mediate some of these effects in the long term, so early identification is of utmost importance (Grace & Sansom, 2003). There is also some evidence which purports that children of anxious or depressed mothers go on to develop these conditions themselves. According to Glover (2016), the rate of mental disorders at 13 years of age for children born to the top 15% most anxious or depressed mothers doubles from around 6% to 12% even after controlling for a range of other causes and effects. Further, if the mother is depressed or anxious both antenatally and postnatally, this risk rises to around 20%. Poor attachment has also been shown to be related to and predictive of poorer infant cognitive outcomes at 18 months (Murray et al., 1996; Robertson & Bowlby, 1952), with some of the strongest effects being seen on cognitive development, such as language skills and intelligence quotient (IQ) (Grace & Sansom, 2003). Early social relations and the development of secure attachment relationships play a vital role in ensuring cognitive and neurobiological health both in childhood and later life (Walsh et al., 2019). Whilst the reasons for this are deeply complex and multifactorial, and children's emotional and cognitive development are also strongly related with socioeconomic factors coupled with wider issues including the couple's relationship and other aspects of parent–child interaction (Glover, 2014); Marryat and Martin (2010) suggest that the children of emotionally well mothers generally have better development in all areas including cognitive than those whose mothers experience PMI. For the children of mothers who experience persistent or repeated mental health problems, this effect was greater still. However, by 36 months, cognitive development was no longer impacted by maternal mood, though the effects on the child's emotional, social and behavioural development were still affected at 46 months and beyond. This suggests that whilst cognitive development may have the tendency to normalise as the child grows, it is the emotional, social and relational effects of maternal mental health problems and poor attachment that are longer lasting.

Transgenerational impact

As has been demonstrated, the effects of maternal mental health problems on the emotional and relational development of the individual child are without question. However, research is also beginning to suggest that the impact may not be limited simply to the individual child but may in fact be transgenerational (Elmadih & Abumadini, 2019). Glover (2016) notes that many women who experience depression during pregnancy and postnatally are survivors of early abuse and are showing symptoms of posttraumatic stress disorder (PTSD) as delineated in Chapter 1. Whilst these conversations can be difficult to have with women and families, as there may be a fear of demonising or inferring blame on the mother, they are important, as she may in fact be experiencing mental health problems relating to her own childhood attachment traumas and will benefit from early treatment and intervention.

Case Study 6.1

Having a mental health disorder that developed in childhood as a result of childhood abuse had an impact on every aspect of my life. When my children arrived, it was clear it would also have a negative impact on those around me, especially the social development of my children.

I would obsess over whether they were breathing right, too hot, too cold, in pain or hungry, to the point where it was taking up most of the day, and I had no energy left for my partner. This contributed to the relationship breakdown that ultimately added trauma to my life and exacerbated symptoms more, as well as left me a single mother and the children no longer living in a traditional family structure with both parents.

As the children became mobile, I would watch them continuously and worry that they would choke on solid food. I would question whether I cut the pieces too big or too small. I would worry about them being out of my care because they were unable to speak and tell me if they were mistreated and would scan their body for any signs that they had been.

I never stopped them from socialising with family or going to playgroup, but I would be walking around in a mental prison with my thoughts turning to my children crying and reaching out for me and I couldn't get to them. They did not suffer directly as I did, but they did suffer indirectly because they had a mother who was on edge and they sensed that.

I then tried to do what I believed was the right thing to do and behaved in the opposite way; I didn't initiate cuddles but let them come to me. If they fell over, I didn't make a big deal of it. This didn't work. The children then got older, and I saw my behaviour rubbing off on them and would see that they did not feel comfortable initiating physical contact with others but would be happy to receive it, which was a relief because I have never been comfortable with physical contact from the sexual abuse and the fear that something bad would happen. Not making a big deal out of accidents worked out favourably though, as they were not needy children and have become grounded, independent young women who now completely understand that for a long time they just had an overprotective mother.

> I would also worry what others were thinking; if my child had bruises, people would be saying I did it. If they got sick, people would believe I made them sick. If the children were not hitting cognitive milestones, people would think I was neglecting them. If my child had a sore bottom from nappy rash, people would think I was molesting them. This would hold an invisible power over me and could have stopped me from seeking medical attention for my children; however, I always put their needs first and would face anything anyone would say, even though it was never said, and I would continue to live in my mental prison.

Warfa et al. (2014) found that not only do insecure attachment and depression in the postpartum period have a common aetiology but that having an insecure attachment style as an adult is a risk factor for developing depressive illness following the birth of the baby. This is because over the lifespan, people have the tendency to maintain consistent strategies for emotional regulation and relating to others. The learned behaviours developed in childhood become the habitual behaviours of adulthood, and these in turn may be passed to future generations. As a predictor of sensitive and responsive caregiving, maternal self-efficacy has also been linked with depressive illness postpartum. Research by Brazeau et al. (2018) found that mothers with higher rates of depression postpartum had lower rates of maternal self-efficacy. In turn, the higher rates of maternal self-efficacy seen in mentally healthy women were linked to more sensitive and responsive caregiving. Low maternal self-efficacy was associated with the woman's own experiences of attachment trauma, childhood maltreatment and the mental health problems of their own mothers. Walsh et al. (2019) support this view in suggesting that early attachment experiences can have profound intergenerational effects through epigenetic mechanisms and their neurobiological consequences – an emerging field in research. It is possible to consider, therefore, that attachment trauma and mental health problems could be passed from generation to generation, being passed from mother to child in an ongoing cycle.

Thus it can be argued that both maternal and paternal mental health matters, as it affects life chances, especially as it is now well established that the quality of the parent–infant relationship is central to the child's social, psychological and cognitive development (Neale, 2017). Parents who are depressed or anxious may find it difficult to form attachment and a meaningful relationship with their baby. There is also sound evidence regarding the deleterious effect on the development of the infant in the presence of parental mental illness (Murray & Cooper, 1997). This is therefore a public health priority due to the consequences of poor PMH on maternal, paternal/partner and child health (Woolhouse et al., 2016). Takács, Smolík, and Putnam (2019) reported that a mother's confidence in her ability to mother her offspring and fulfil her parenting role may be affected by the woman's experience of parenting an infant that is perceived as difficult as well as the woman's depressive symptomatology, especially during the first year of the infant's life.

Stress and anxiety

It is reported that marked levels of stress and anxiety as a consequence of poor parenting skills or suboptimal parenting in the formative years of a child's life can markedly disturb cognitive development by disrupting the evolving nervous system as well as the stress hormone regulatory system (Barlow et al., 2015; Gerhardt, 2004; Swain, 2011). As discussed in parent–infant relationship section of the chapter, it is evident that parental ability to regulate their child's emotional state plays a pivotal role in helping children to develop strategies for self-regulation (Barlow et al., 2015). Gerhardt (2004) argued that the ramifications of the inability of parents, the primary caregivers, to respond appropriately to the needs of their infant can lead to a harmful effect at the neurochemical level due to prolonged increase of cortisol levels on the infant. This conclusion of Gerhardt (2004) was based on the evidence reviewed, which highlighted prolonged levels of cortisol in early childhood have consequences for the not yet fully developed nervous system. This is significant in terms of how the infant tolerates stress later in life via the hypothalamic-pituitary-adrenal axis and prefrontal cortex. Barlow et al. (2015) state that the net result of such adversity can be detrimental in terms of how young children respond to threat. Children who develop insecure relationships with their parents may develop maladaptive behaviour, and it could affect the way they respond to threat and their future relationships with their peers and significant others in later life, as well as increase their susceptibility to mental illness and other morbidity (Barlow et al., 2015; Glover, 2014; Skovgaard, 2010).

Fatherhood

The literature is replete with information around the transition to motherhood, but this is often to the neglect of fathers. Fatherhood, like motherhood, is a social construct largely shaped and influenced by social mores and cultural context in which men are socialised (Shorey & Ang, 2019). In contemporary Western societies, the modern-day father is not a homogeneous group. Fathers come in various forms. Fathers can be married or single; be stay at home dads who are employed or unemployed; be an adoptive, foster or stepfather and be either gay, heterosexual or non-binary. More importantly, fathers have a pivotal role to play in childrearing and are very capable care providers in the early years and beyond towards children's psychosocial and physical wellbeing. A growing body of evidence from psychological research within cross-cultural settings and a variety of ethnic backgrounds conclude that fathers' affection, support and nurturing of children play a central role to a child's social and emotional wellbeing (Eskandri et al., 2016; Neale, 2017; Glasser & Lerner-Geva, 2019). The following case study provides an insight into one father's transition to fatherhood.

Case Study 6.2   Transition to fatherhood: A dad's journey

Preparation for becoming a father

When thinking about the whole process of becoming a father, I have to go back to life before children and remember what this life was like. I was happy within my relationship and liked the life we had together. Although the idea of having children was not something I had a strong desire for, I didn't rule it out. However, my partner felt very differently, and this was something totally essential for her. Having been in a previous relationship that hadn't worked out, my main concern was maintaining the aspects of our relationship that I cherished most and wondered how this would change with children in our lives. How would I squeeze this new person into my already busy work life, and would I really be able to give enough of my time and myself to this new person? All these questions and more swirled around my mind, my partner convinced me that we could have both a loving relationship with time for each other, coupled with the fulfilling experience that children bring.

So the decision was made, with an indecisive me, feeling that I was walking away from a comfortable life and into the unknown. My partner, however, had total conviction, assuring me that the new addition would work around us. What could go wrong?

The start of the pregnancy was slightly numbing for me, as now after all the talk it was actually happening. Normal life was put on hold a bit as we both adapted to a new pattern for the next 9 months. It wasn't me having the baby, but the due date felt like an exam scheduled months in advance; although it was a long time off, at some point I would have to face that day. This prospect didn't seem to concern my partner, but it made me feel extremely apprehensive for my soul mate.

I remember the feeling after seeing the baby during the hospital scan, which didn't feel particularly emotional or meaningful for either of us. I felt unconnected at that point and wondered if I would still feel like

(Continued)

this when the reality of the birth happened. It was these moments that made me feel more like a bystander just watching things unfold. I remember asking my partner, 'What if I didn't have any connection with our child when it was born?' But she just laughed and said not to worry.

As I was watching someone else do all the work during the course of the pregnancy, I found myself throwing my energy into researching novel morning sickness cures, best foods for babies and the equipment we needed for this new addition. I even started looking at schools way too early!

Decorating the house was something else I really got into while pre-paring for the big day. In my mind, I was preparing a safe loving environ-ment, and imagining the newborn baby in this lovingly decorated home gave me a warm, loving feeling inside.

I have a happy memory towards the end of the pregnancy of the ante-natal classes that we did with friends that gave me a bit of reassurance of how to tackle what was around the corner, and I felt more secure in my preparedness.

The birth itself was a great experience, nervous excitement going into labour and the relief after a safe birth. During the birth, I felt connected with my partner; we were a team, and I was the support coach in charge of hand-holding, breathing in time together and sharing snacks. I just wanted to live as much of it as I could with her, so I could take her pain away. My most vivid memory was seeing my daughter 15 minutes after she was born, lying under the heat lamp in the hospital. Her eyes were wide open, and as I looked into those beautiful eyes, I felt drawn in as if there were a universe of feelings behind them. At that moment I was no longer a bystander. I said to myself I was going to look after her for the rest of my life, and I meant it.

After the birth…my new life!

For the first few months we had a very simple life together. It was almost a cocoon-like feeling of our new family unit and was very pleasant.

From a practical point of view, my partner decided that we should both be able to look after the baby if she wasn't around in case of an emergency or she just wanted time away with friends. I learnt how to look after my daughter, so if my other half was out, I could cope. We took turns looking after the baby; if one of us was up in the night we made sure the other one was sleeping. Although this gave me more responsibility, it also helped me with the bonding experience of getting to know my child and ease the pressure from our relationship by giving my partner time out – after all, a more rested mum is more pleasant to be around. I do believe that, as a father, just like in life, if you put more into something you get more out. You become more of a teammate with your partner so there's less chance of feeling isolated.

So how has the indecisive father that didn't have a strong drive to become a parent adapted? Largely okay. My world is not just about me now, and that sense of responsibility has developed me as a person. Sometimes when the pressure of work and family life collide at the same time, it's hard not to feel resentment, as I was assured by my partner that children wouldn't get in the way of my work. However, with my level of involvement, this is impossible. As well, when I'm making an effort to lighten her workload for the life she wanted, there are times when I feel she's putting more energy into her friends than into me. However this is true of any relationship; it's something you have to work at, and the pressure from children just adds to the challenge. When I do feel resentment, I find that taking myself back to that night when I first connected with my daughter reminds me of what it's all about.

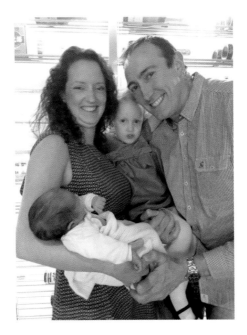

Image 6.2 Thanks to Paul Tolley, Amy and children Charlotte and baby Darcey.

Fathers/partners and perinatal mental health

While the bulk of literature on parenting focuses on the mother's role and care, research increasingly examines the highly significant and over-looked role of fathers. Hanley and Williams (2017) attest that for decades the mental health of new fathers in the perinatal period has been overlooked and neglected. Nonetheless, although under-researched, there is now growing evidence of the mental health problems expectant and new fathers encounter (Baldwin & Bick, 2017; Baldwin et al., 2018; NHS England, 2019). An improved picture is beginning to emerge with more awareness, education and understanding of this under-investigated subject. This means that midwives and allied health care professionals have a re-sponsibility to male partners of pregnant women and new mothers who are mentally unwell to ensure they are not left to flounder and suffer in silence.

A systemic review by Baldwin et al. (2018) underscored three main factors that impact first-time fathers' mental health and wellbeing as they make their transition to fatherhood. They are:

* the formation of fatherhood identity,
* competing challenges of the new role fatherhood brings and
* negative feelings and fears the new role of fatherhood imposes on self and lifestyle.

Additionally, Baldwin and Bick (2017) explained that there are a num-ber of common risk factors for paternal anxiety and depression during the transition to fatherhood as delineated by Box 6.1.

Paternal depression is a factor related to children's emotional, behavioural and social function in the early years (Glasser & Lerner-Geva, 2019). This is a common feature during the transition to parenthood, as reported by Cameron, Sedov, and Tomfohr-Madsen (2016), who

---

Box 6.1 Some common risk factors for paternal anxiety and depression during the transition to fatherhood

* Relationship discord/poor relationship satisfaction
* Socioeconomic difficulties such as unemployment and social deprivation
* Young adolescent male/immaturity
* Unplanned pregnancy
* History of depression
* Lack of or poor quality social and emotional support
* Having a partner with mental illness

Adapted from Baldwin S., Bick D. (2017). First-time fathers' needs and experienc-es of transition to fatherhood in relation to their mental health and wellbeing: a qualitative systematic review protocol. JBI Database System Rev Implement Rep; 15(3):647–56.

highlight a prevalence rate of paternal depression to be around 8% but cautioned that when examining the evidence, there are a number of variables at play that often result in marked heterogeneity in rates based on assessment tool, study location and rates of maternal depression. This is noted by the Glasser and Lerner-Geva (2019) literature review reflecting a prevalence of paternal depression between 2% and 8%. NHS England (2019) identified that the prevalence rates for anxiety and depression symptoms in men in the first 6 months of an infant's life is about 1 in 10.

Social support

During periods of stress and anxiety such as the transition to parenthood, supportive and compassionate care from midwives will not only help promote self-efficacy and emotional wellbeing for parents as they adapt to their parenting role but also aid in the amelioration of threatened psychological morbidity postpartum (Bouchard, 2014; NICE, 2014, 2018; Oakley et al., 1996). Midwives are well placed to be cognisant of the significance of social support and the contribution and part played by friends, families, the wider community and health care professionals in augmenting parental self-efficacy and promoting health and wellbeing, especially mental health in the early postpartum period (Coates & Foureur, 2019; Sandall et al., 2016).

Social support refers to empathy relations, emotional support, intelligence support and economic or financial support (Raynor, 2020). During periods of stress, supportive and holistic care from midwives will not only assist in promoting emotional wellbeing of parents but will also help to ameliorate threatened psychological morbidity postpartum (NHS England, 2019; NICE, 2014, 2018). Parents who are socially isolated, feel marginalised in society or who have poor socioeconomic means are particularly vulnerable to PMH problems and will need additional help and support. Midwives should be alert to families who are displaced from their communities (e.g. asylum seekers, refugees, families from minority ethnic groups who do not speak English) and who may have difficulties accessing health care and understanding and navigating the health care system (Knight et al., 2019).

Social support is a form of psychological therapy. Indeed for most mothers and fathers with mild depressive illness or emotional distress and difficulties adjusting to their parenting role, extra time given by the midwife or health visitor, popularly regarded as 'the listening visit', will be effective (NICE, 2014, 2018). Particularly for parents with more persistent states associated with high levels of anxiety, NICE (2014, 2018) states that brief cognitive behavioural therapy (CBT) and interpersonal psychotherapy are as effective as pharmacological treatment (e.g. antidepressants; see Chapter 3). Such psychological therapies often confer additional benefits in terms of improving the parent–infant relationship and overall satisfaction with the parenting role (NICE, 2014, 2018; Raynor, 2020).

Lack of social support, particularly when combined with adversity, severe and multiple social inequalities and major life events, has long been implicated in the aetiology of mild to moderate depressive illness (NICE, 2014, 2018). Social support includes not only practical assistance and advice but also an emotional confidant, close friends, family and communities who improve the locus of control, self-efficacy and self-esteem. There is also evidence that community services that are underpinned by social support theory can have a beneficial effect on the parent–infant relationship and wellbeing, which might be instrumental in helping to alleviate mild depressive symptomatology postpartum (Barlow et al., 2015).

Supporting fathers

Although NICE (2014, 2018) identified the value of social support in promoting mental health and wellbeing for mothers, the needs of fathers are not addressed. Nonetheless, there is help and support available to men to assist in their adjustment to fatherhood. It is important that information is provided to meet individual needs. Table 6.1 highlights areas of support for fathers. Baldwin et al. (2018) assert that the significant restrictions in roles and upheavals bring about changes that a number of fathers do not bargain for (see Case Study 6.2). Coupled with this is the necessary adjustments in lifestyle that may leave many new fathers feeling worried and stressed. To help ameliorate these feelings, some fathers reportedly employed denial tactics or means of escapism pursuits such as engaging in longer working hours, listening to music and smoking. The information needs and support men wanted related to better guidance to prepare for their new role as fathers as well as the reality and practicalities involved in becoming a father, including how this might disrupt and have an impact on the intimate relationship with their partner. The support of midwives during this critical period in men's lives would help to break down barriers, generate useful resources, create networking opportunities and fulfil the information needs of expectant fathers, thus helping to make a positive difference in the adjustment and mental wellbeing in new fathers.

Table 6.1: Supporting fathers

Preconception education
The importance of optimal health and family planning should be explained not only to girls/women but also to boys/men. Information should be provided about strategies to ensure optimal health by examining the health implications of lifestyle activities such as exercise, diet, smoking, alcohol, drugs misuse, stress/anxiety and wider mental health issues.

Meeting fathers' information needs
Research by Teague and Shatte (2018) demonstrated that men use technology and web-based communities to share the joys and challenges of the fatherhood experience. This is supported by Fletcher et al. (2019), who evaluated using a Short Message Service (SMS) text-based approach to support fathers.

Relationship
The range of emotions involved in the transition to parenthood should be explained including role changes, the disruption that a new baby brings in a household (especially if the man is new to fatherhood), common stress factors, such as changes to financial status, role changes/role conflict, disrupted sleep, sense of social isolation from friends and relationship discord.

Parent education classes for expectant fathers
This can be achieved through a variety of different approaches such as peer support sessions, digital platforms that encourage live chats among new fathers or face-to-face classes specifically for men.

Creating more family-friendly spaces within the hospital environment
Because the majority of births in the UK now take place within a hospital setting, there is a push for such institutional settings to enable fathers to stay overnight with their partners and new babies if that is their wish, rather than literally getting shut out once the prescribed visiting hours end. This approach will help to positively foster and nurture the father–infant relationship.

Fathers with mental health problems
The NHS Long Term Plan (NHS England, 2019) emphasises the importance of the fathering role and the capacity of PMH services to provide peer support, relationship talking therapies/behavioural therapy for couples plus other family and parenting interventions. These interventions might include parenting skills and other common mental health condition treatments such as Improving Access to Psychological Therapies (IAPT).

Conclusion

In understanding the importance of the parent–infant relationship to child development, midwives are well placed to respond to the PMH needs of women, their partners and the families for whom they care. This chapter has shone a spotlight on the fact that PMH problems not only affect women, their partners, their families and wider society but also impact the psychosocial, physical and emotional development of infants through the parent–infant interactions and relationship. The negative outcomes for an infant, it has been argued, can be protracted and act as a continuum throughout the formative years of childhood and adulthood. The intergenerational implications of this have also been highlighted. Social support has an important role to play, as it acts as a buffer and contributes to the positive adjustment to parenthood and a more harmonious relationship between parents and their offspring.

Practice Learning Points

- The quality of the parent–infant attachment and general relationship in the early years is a prevailing predictor of an infant's subsequent social, emotional and cognitive development.
- Poor maternal mental health can have a detrimental effect on the maternal–infant bond.
- Disrupted maternal–infant bonding can create attachment trauma and result in insecure attachment in the child.
- Paternal depression is a factor related to children's emotional, behavioural and social function in the early years.
- Increasingly, research is examining the highly significant and overlooked role of fathers and their contribution to childrearing.
- The children of mothers experiencing mental health problems are 5.4 times more likely to display signs of insecure attachment.
- The effects of insecure attachment for the child can include problems with emotional regulation, cognitive development, future relationships and mental health problems.
- Mothers experiencing depression postpartum are more likely to have experienced attachment traumas themselves.
- Attachment trauma can be seen as both a result of and a cause of depression in the postpartum period.
- The effects of attachment trauma and mental health problems may be transgenerational.

POINTS FOR REFLECTION

- *What do you understand by the term parent–infant attachment?*
- *How would you as a midwife apply knowledge of attachment theory to promote and encourage close and loving relationships between new parents and their babies?*
- *Why is the parent–infant relationship of such significance to child development?*

Acknowledgements

Many thanks to Sherry Whibley, Paul Tolley and family who shared their personal experience of parenthood in order that others can learn from their story.

References

Ainsworth, M. D. S., & Bell, S. M. (1970). Attachment, exploration, and separation: Illustrated by the behavior of one-year-olds in a strange situation. *Child Development*, 41, 49–67. Retrieved May 06, 2020 from https://www.jstor.org/stable/1127388?seq=1.

Ainsworth, M. S. (1979). Infant–mother attachment. *American Psychologist*, 34(10), 932–937. https://doi.org/10.1037/0003-066X.34.10.932.

Atkinson, L., Paglia, A., Coolbear, J., et al. (2000). Attachment security: A meta-analysis of maternal mental health correlates. *Clinical Psychology Review*, 20, 1019–1040. Retrieved May 05, 2020 from https://www.ncbi.nlm.nih.gov/pubmed/11098398.

Ayers, S., & Sawyer, A. (2019). The impact of birth on women's health and wellbeing. In O. T. Ben-Ari (Ed.), *Pathways and barriers to parenthood* (pp. 199–218). Cham: Springer.

Baldwin, S., & Bick, D. (2017). First-time fathers' needs and experiences of transition to fatherhood in relation to their mental health and wellbeing: A qualitative systematic review protocol. *Joanna Briggs Institute (JBI) Database of Systematic Reviews and Implementation Reports*, 15(3), 647–656.

Baldwin, S., Malone, M., Sandall, J., & Bick, D. (2018). Mental health and wellbeing during the transition to fatherhood: A systematic review of first time fathers' experiences. *Joanna Briggs Institute (JBI) Database of Systematic Reviews and Implementation Reports*, 16(11), 2118–2191.

Barlow, J., Bennett, C., Midgley, N., Larkin, S. K., & Wei, Y. (2015). Parent–infant psychotherapy for improving parental and infant mental health. *Cochrane Database of Systematic Reviews*; 1: CD010534. https://doi.org/10.1002/14651858.CD010534.pub2. PMID: 25569177.

Bouchard, G. (2014). The quality of the parenting alliance during the transition to parenthood. *Canadian Journal of Behavioural Science*, 46(1), 20–28.

Bowlby, J. (1958). The nature of the child's tie to his mother. *International Journal of Psychoanalysis*, 39, 350–371. Retrieved May 05, 2020 from https://pubmed.ncbi.nlm.nih.gov/13610508/.

Bowlby, J. (1969). Attachment. *Attachment and loss: Vol. 1. Loss*. New York: Basic Books.

Bowlby, J., Ainsworth, M., Boston, M., & Rosenbluth, D. (1956). The effects of mother-child separation: A follow-up study. *British Journal of Medical Psychology*, 29, 211–224. Retrieved May 05, 2020 from https://www.ncbi.nlm.nih.gov/pubmed/13355922.

Brazeau, N., Reisz, S., Jacobvitz, D., & George, C. (2018). Understanding the connection between attachment trauma and maternal self-efficacy in depressed mothers. *Infant Mental Health Journal*, 39(1), 30–43. https://doi.org/10.1002/imhj.21692.

Bretherton, I. (1992). The origins of attachment theory: John Bowlby and Mary Ainsworth. *Journal of Developmental Psychology*, 28(5), 759–775.

Cameron, E. E., Sedov, I. D., & Tomfohr-Madsen, L. M. (2016). Prevalence of paternal depression in pregnancy and the postpartum: An updated meta-analysis. *Journal of Affective Disorders*, 206, 189–203. https://doi.org/10.1016/j.jad.2016.07.044.

Coates, D., & Foureur, M. (2019). The role and competence of midwives in supporting women with mental health concerns during the perinatal period: A scoping review. *Health & Social Care in the Community*, 27(4), e389–e405. https://doi.org/10.1111/hsc.12740.

Dollard, J., & Miller, N. E. (1950). *Personality and psychotherapy*. New York: McGraw-Hill.

Elmadih, A., & Abumadini, M. (2019). Epigenetic transmission of maternal behavior: Impact on the neurobiological system of healthy mothers. *Saudi Journal of Medicine and Medical Sciences*, 7(1), 3–8. https://doi.org/10.4103/sjmms.sjmms_163_17.

Eskandri, N., Simbar, M., Vedadhir, A., & Baghestani, A. R. (2016). Paternal adaptation in first-time fathers: A phenomenological study. *Journal of Reproductive and Infant Psychology*, 2017 Feb;35(1):53–64. https://doi.org/10.1080/02646838.2016.1233480. Epub 2016 Oct 28. PMID: 29517289.

Fletcher, R., Knight, T., Macdonald, J. A., & St George, A. (2019). Process evaluation of text-based support for fathers during the transition to fatherhood (SMS4dads): Mechanisms of impact. *BMC Psychology*, 7, 63. https://doi.org/10.1186/s40359-019-0338.

Gerhardt, S. (2004). *Why love matters: How affection shapes a baby's brain*. New York: Routledge/Taylor and Francis Group.

Gillath, O., Karantzas, G. C., & Fraley, R. C. (2016). *Adult attachment: A concise introduction to theory and research* (1st ed.). London: Academic Press.

Glasser, S., & Lerner-Geva, L. (2019). Focus on fathers: Paternal depression in the perinatal period. *Perspect Public Health*, 139(4), 195–198. https://doi.org/10.1177/1757913918790597. Epub 2018 Jul 25. PMID: 30044191.

Glover, V. (2014). Maternal depression, anxiety and stress during pregnancy and child outcome; what needs to be done? *Best Practice and Research in Clinical Obstetrics and Gynaecology*, 28(1), 25–35.

Glover, V. (2016). Perinatal mental health, attachment and the development of the child. Presentation to the early years, parenting and relationships conference. *Early Intervention Foundation*. https://www.eif.org.uk.

Grace, S. L., & Sansom, S. (2003). The effect of postpartum depression on the mother-infant relationship and child growth and development. In D. E. Stewart, E. Robertson, & C. L. Dennis (Eds.), *Postpartum depression: Literature review of risk factors and interventions*. Department of Mental Health and Substance Abuse. World Health Organization, 197–251.

Hanley, J., & Williams, M. (2017). Assessing and managing paternal mental health issues. *Nursing Times (online)*, 114(12), 26–29.

On behalf of MBRRACE-UK, Knight, M., Bunch, K., & Tuffnell, D. (Eds.), (2019). *Saving lives, improving mothers' care – Lessons learned to inform maternity care from the UK and Ireland Confidential Enquiries into Maternal Deaths and Morbidity 2015–17*. Oxford: National Perinatal Epidemiology Unit, University of Oxford.

Marryat, L., & Martin, C. (2010). *Growing up in Scotland: Maternal mental health and its impact on child behaviour and development.* Edinburgh: Scottish Centre for Social Research.

Mikulincer, M., & Shaver, P. R. (2012). An attachment perspective on psychopathology. *World Psychiatry: Official Journal of the World Psychiatric Association (WPA)*, 11, 11–15.

Murray, L., & Cooper, P. J. (1997). Effects of postnatal depression on infant development. *Archives of Disease in Childhood*, 77(2), 99–101.

Murray, L., Fiori-Cowley, A., Hooper, R., & Cooper, P. (1996). The impact of postnatal depression and associated adversity on early mother-infant interactions and later infant outcome. *Child Development*, 67(5), 1891–1914. Retrieved May 07, 2020 from https://www.ncbi.nlm.nih.gov/pubmed/9022253.

National Institute for Health and Care Excellence (NICE). (2014). *Antenatal and postnatal mental health. The NICE guidelines on clinical management and service guidance (updated EDN, CG 192).* London: NICE. Updated 2018. Retrieved May 02, 2020 from https://www.nice.org.uk/guidance/cg192/evidence/full-guideline-pdf-4840896925.

Neale, D. (2017). The psychology of babies: How relationships support development from birth to two. *Journal of Reproductive and Infant Psychology*, 35(1), 103–104. https://doi.org/10.1080/02646838.2016.1186267.

NHS England. (2016a). National Maternity Review – Better Births: Improving outcomes of maternity services in England, a five year forward view for maternity care. https://www.england.nhs.uk/wp-content/uploads/2016/02/national-maternity-review-report.pdf

NHS England. (2016b). *A five year forward view for mental health: Report from the independent Mental Health Taskforce to the NHS in England.* Retrieved May 01, 2020 from https://www.england.nhs.uk/wp-content/uploads/2016/02/Mental-Health-Taskforce-FYFV-final.pdf

NHS England. (2019). *The NHS Long Term Plan.* Retrieved April 29, 2020 from https://www.longtermplan.nhs.uk/wp-content/uploads/2019/08/nhs-long-term-plan-version-1.2.pdf

Oakley, A., Hickey, D., Rajan, L., & Rigby, A. S. (1996). Social support in pregnancy: Does it have long-term effects? *Journal of Reproductive and Infant Psychology*, 14(1), 7–22. https://doi.org/10.1080/02646839608405855.

Raynor, M. D. (2020). Perinatal mental health. In J. E. M. Marshall & M. D. Raynor (Eds.), *Myles textbook for midwives* (17th ed.). Edinburgh: Churchill Livingstone. Chap. 30.

Rholes, W. S., & Paetzold, R. L. (2019). Attachment and the transition to parenthood. In O. T. Ben-Ari (Ed.), *Pathways and barriers to parenthood* (pp. 291–303). Cham: Springer.

Robertson, J., & Bowlby, J. (1952). Responses of young children to separation from their mothers II: Observations of the sequences of response of children aged 18 to 24 months during the course of separation. *Courrier du Centre International de l'Enfance, 2*, 131–142.

Rutter, M. (1979). Maternal deprivation, 1972–1978: New findings, new concepts, new approaches. *Child Development, 50*(2), 283–305. Retrieved May 05, 2020 from https://pubmed.ncbi.nlm.nih.gov/114367/.

Sandall, J., Soltani, H., Gates, S., Shennan, A., & Devane, D. (2016). Midwife-led continuity models versus other models of care for childbearing women. *Cochrane Database of Systematic Reviews*, Apr 28;4:CD004667. https://doi.org/10.1002/14651858.CD004667.pub5. PMID: 27121907.

Schaffer, H. R., & Emerson, P. E. (1964). The development of social attachments in infancy. *Monographs of the Society for Research in Child Development, 29*(3), 1–77. JSTOR, www.jstor.org/stable/1165727. Retrieved May 05, 2020 from https://europepmc.org/article/med/14151332.

Shorey, S., & Ang, L. (2019). Experiences, needs, and perceptions of paternal involvement during the first year after their infants' birth: A meta-synthesis. *PLoS One, 14*(1), e0210388. https://doi.org/10.1371/journal.pone.0210388.

Skovgaard, A. M. (2010). Mental health problems and psychopathology in infancy and early childhood: An epidemiological study. *Danish medical bulletin, 57*, 1–30.

Swain, J. E. (2011). Becoming a parent – biobehavioral and brain science perspectives. *Current Problems in Pediatric and Adolescent Health Care, 41*, 192–196. https://doi.org/10.1016/j.cppeds.2011.02.004.

Takács, L., Smolík, F., & Putnam, S. (2019). Assessing longitudinal pathways between maternal depressive symptoms, parenting self-esteem and infant temperament (eCollection). *PLoS One, 14*(8), e0220633. https://doi.org/10.1371/journal.pone.0220633.

Teague, S. J., & Shatte, A. B. (2018). Exploring the transition to fatherhood: Feasibility study using social media and machine learning. *JMIR Pediatrics and Parenting, 1*(2), e12371. https://doi.org/10.2196/12371.

Toth, S. L., Rogosch, F. A., Sturge-Apple, M., & Cicchetti, D. (2009). Maternal depression, children's attachment security, and representational development: An organizational perspective. *Journal of Child Development, 80*(1), 192–208. https://doi.org/10.1111/j.1467-8624.2008.01254.x.

UNICEF. (2013). *The evidence and rationale for the UNICEF UK Baby Friendly Initiative standards*. London: UNICEF UK.

UNICEF. (2019). *Guide to the UNICEF UK Baby Friendly Initiative university standards*. London: UNICEF UK.

Walsh, E., Blake, Y., Donati, A., Stoop, R., & von Gunten, A. (2019). Early secure attachment as a protective factor against later cognitive decline and dementia. *Frontiers in Aging Neuroscience, 11*:161. https://doi.org/10.3389/fnagi.2019.00161.

Warfa, N., Harper, M., Nicolais, G., & Bhui, K. (2014). Adult attachment style as a risk factor for maternal postnatal depression: a systematic review.

BMC Psychology, Dec 18;2(1):56. https://doi.org/10.1186/s40359-014-0056-x. PMID: 25926974; PMCID: PMC4407393.

Woolhouse, H., Gartland, D., Mensah, F., et al. (2016). Maternal depression from pregnancy to 4 years postpartum and emotional/behavioural difficulties in children: Results from a prospective pregnancy cohort study. *Archives of Women's Mental Health*, 19(1), 141–151.

World Health Organization (WHO). (2004). *The importance of caregiver-child interactions for the survival and healthy development of young children: A review.* Retrieved May 05, 2020 from https://www.who.int/maternal_child_adoles centdocuments/924159134X/en/

World Health Organization (WHO). (2015). *Thinking healthy: A manual for psychological management of perinatal depression.* Retrieved May 05, 2020 from https://www.who.int/mental_health/maternal-child/thinking_healthy/en/

Suggested further reading

McNamara, J., Townsend, M. L., & Herbert, J. S. (2019). A systemic review of maternal wellbeing and its relationship with maternal fetal attachment and early postpartum bonding. *PLoS One*, 14(7), e0220032. https://doi.org/10.1371/journal.pone.0220032.

An informative systematic review that synthesizes the published literature to determine the nature of the relationship between a pregnant woman's psychological wellbeing and the development of maternal–fetal attachment. This spans the antenatal and early postnatal period where the authors aimed to identify key recommendations for future research and clinical practice.

Lehnig, F., Nagl, M., Stepan, H., Wagner, B. (2019). Associations of postpartum mother-infant bonding with maternal childhood maltreatment and postpartum mental health: A cross-sectional study. *BMC Pregnancy & Childbirth*, 19, 278. https://doi.org/10.1186/s12884-019-2426-0.

This article provides an overview of traumatic stress sequelae of childhood maltreatment and adversity in the context of the mother–infant relationship.

van Rosmalen, L., van der Veer, R., & van der Horst, F. C. (2020). The nature of love: Harlow, Bowlby and Bettelheim on affectionless mothers. *History of Psychiatry*, 31(2), 227–231. https://doi.org/10.1177/0957154X19898997.

This article provides a useful critique of some of the historical psychological research that has shaped our understanding of the parent–infant dynamic relationship.

World Health Organization: https://www.who.int.

e-Learning programmes on perinatal mental health available to midwives

https://www.e-lfh.org.uk/programmes/perinatal-mental-health: This consists of three modules primarily aimed at health visitors but has some useful information and video clips.

https://www.ilearn.rcm.org.uk: provided by the Royal College of Midwives.

CHAPTER 7

The perinatal mental health midwifery toolkit

Michelle Anderson and Anna-Marie Madeley

Part 1: The role of the midwife

The role of the midwife is constantly developing and expanding. The autonomy of midwifery practice requires complex decision making in relation to women-centred care. The ability to identify deviations from normal physiology is crucial when considering plans of care for women and their families. Detecting changes in normal physical parameters is relatively straightforward, for example, a sustained blood pressure reading of 164/98 mmHg requires urgent investigation, or a low haemoglobin level can be easily detected through a blood test and treated appropriately with iron supplementation. However, changes to mental health can be much more difficult to identify, leaving women to fall through the gap between maternity and mental health services (Coates & Foureur, 2019).

As discussed in previous chapters, perinatal mental illness (PMI) is not uncommon, and all midwives should have at least basic knowledge of mental health conditions that may affect women during pregnancy and beyond. Yet, knowledge itself is not enough to equip midwives to support women who are affected by PMI, for it is only one cog in the ever-turning complex wheel of mental health. As such, a pragmatic as well as theoretical approach is needed to support the care of women experiencing PMI.

Understanding perinatal mental illness

Mental health is complex, and for those affected by mental illness, there is usually not one definitive reason for the diagnosis. However, there are well-documented risk factors that increase the likelihood of developing PMI. Circumstances dominated by poverty and socioeconomic disadvantage are contributing factors towards poor mental health (The Woman's Mental Health Taskforce, 2018), as are a family history of poor mental health, drug and alcohol abuse and a history of childhood and sexual abuse (PHE, 2019).

Consideration should also be given to black, Asian and minority ethnic (BAME) women who may face additional barriers to accessing mental health support (The Woman's Mental Health Taskforce, 2018). It is likely that this is a contributing factor as to why black women still have more than five times the risk of dying in pregnancy or up to 6 weeks postpartum compared with white women (MBRRACE, 2019). This suggestion is worth further analysis because of the 549 women who died in the United Kingdom between 2015 and 2017, 70% were from Asia and Africa, and 20% of women who died were known to social services, suggesting higher levels of vulnerability (MBRRACE, 2019). Although mental health was not a predominant factor in the cause of death for the majority of women, it may well have been a contributing variable.

The consequences of mental health illness can be devastating. Suicide was found to be the second-largest cause of maternal deaths between 2015 and 2017 within 42 days postnatally (MBRRACE, 2019). What circumstances lead a new mother to end her life? The question is poignant and one that remains difficult to answer.

Severe mental disorder after birth and a history of self-harm are strongly associated with increased risk of suicide in the postpartum year (Lysell et al., 2018). Suicidal ideations and acts are also associated with adjustment disorder, depressive episodes and anxiety rather than a psychotic disorder (Doherty, Crudden, Jabbar, Sheehan, & Casey, 2019; Grigoriasdis et al., 2017; Kendig et al., 2017). Furthermore, one Canadian study found many of the women who ended their lives had contact with mental health services in the year before suicide (Grigoriasdis et al., 2017).

Women with severe mental illness may be more at risk of relapse during pregnancy, and it is important that these women continue to take their medications. Women with bipolar 1, for example, are at particular risk of postpartum psychosis, but postpartum psychosis can occur in women without any previous history of mental illness (NICE, 2014).

For some women, the change to mental illness may be more subtle. A proportion of women may experience increased anxiety or develop depression during pregnancy for the first time. In fact, these are the two most common conditions that can manifest during the antenatal period (NICE, 2014). In some cases, women do not always disclose when their mental health deteriorates. Reasons for this include feeling unprepared for changes to mental health when coping with the transition and adaptation to motherhood; finding it difficult to differentiate between 'normal' feelings, behaviours and tiredness and symptoms requiring further support; simply not wanting to 'make a fuss'; and worrying about the stigma associated with mental illness and seeking help (Khan, 2015).

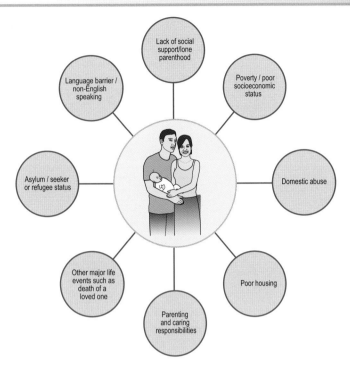

Fig 7.1 Vulnerability factors and mental health.

It is imperative, therefore, that mental illness and deteriorating mental health is identified as soon as possible. Better Births and the roll out of continuity of carer service models have contributed to increased support for women with perinatal mental health issues (The Maternity Transformation Programme, 2020). Many NHS trusts offer continuity of carer models for vulnerable women and women with mental illness. These models are beneficial and have been shown to engage women with treatment for their mental health and increase support to access mental health services, enabling women to build a longer-term relationship of mutual trust and respect with the midwife, who can support women to make informed decisions (Marks, Siddle, & Warwick, 2003; The Maternity Transformation Programme, 2020).

Reflection from Stephanie (vulnerable women's team midwife at The Royal Free NHS FT)

The most satisfying aspect of care is being able to build relationships with women and their families to support their individual needs. I believe that working with women who experience complex social and/or psychological challenges builds resilience and professional growth. There are women who have had adverse childhood experiences (ACEs), personality disorders, anti-social behaviour, high levels of anxiety and much more. Their experiences and current challenges can either support relationship-building or be a barrier.

A proportion of women are under specialised care due to substance use or current social care involvement and do not wish to be with a vulnerable women's team. They report that this is because they feel judged or singled out by the system. Many of these women respond with verbal aggression, dismissive behaviour or non-engagement.

As midwives, we all strive to build relationships with women and give the best care possible. When women choose not to engage, it can be frustrating, emotionally draining and time consuming. One booking appointment, antenatal appointment, postnatal appointment or phone call could unexpectedly take up half a day with referrals, follow ups, documentation and discussion on case management.

Although our organisational skills are highly proficient, the day rarely goes as planned. It may start with a call from triage about a woman with suicidal ideation, an impromptu text from a client needing domestic violence support, urgent calls from social care about new or escalating concerns or a call from the birth centre or delivery suite to provide intrapartum care. There are several things that will require a reprioritisation of tasks, which leaves two options: Move everything else to another day or once again work very late, both of which have their challenges. Moving appointments sometimes means that continuity is interrupted, which may not be beneficial to specific women and also adds pressure to other members of the team with their own increasing caseload.

However, being in a team of professionals with good relationships and trust really helps. I fully appreciate the value of every team member and I know I could not do my job successfully without every single one of them. Between us we have a vast range of strengths, knowledge and experience. We are always learning something new from each other and recharging each other's metaphorical batteries. In the wider team, the safeguarding advisors are available to provide supervision and play a large part in our professional development as specialist midwives. Fresh eyes on a case from someone with more experience or a different perspective is so valuable in the management and sometimes decision to reallocate cases with developing complexity.

Practice learning point

- *Keep reflecting. There is something new to learn from each case, whether challenging or positive.*
- *Ask for help. Safeguarding supervision, extra training, multi-professional advice and others in your team have a vast range of knowledge and perspective to support you and your development.*
- *Trust your team. If you trust each other, you not only learn from each other but also feel able to have your days off and feel confident that all women are well supported.*
- *Take care of yourself because you cannot help anyone else if you are not OK.*

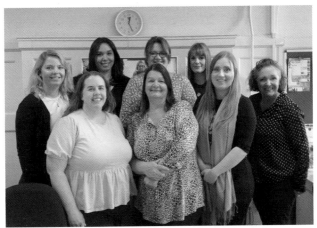

Fig 7.2 The Acacia Team for Vulnerable Women (Barnet Hospital).

The midwifery perinatal mental illness toolkit

Many midwives who are not specialists in the role find the topic of mental health difficult to approach with women. This is often for a myriad of reasons such as a lack of confidence, skills and knowledge or predominantly inadequate training provision (Coates & Foureur, 2019). However, with improved training, midwives can play a crucial part in enhancing perinatal mental health care by developing relationships that create safe conditions for disclosure, providing information on symptoms of PMI to the women and her wider support network and having knowledge on appropriate resources and referral pathways that may benefit the woman and her family (Viveiros & Darling, 2018).

Practice learning point

Key factors in creating a safe environment for disclosure:

- *Practise good communication*
- *Give the woman time and space to build a trusting relationship*
- *Acknowledge that the woman might not disclose PMI at the first appointment*
- *Exhibit professional curiosity by:*
  - *Exploration and reading between the lines*
  - *Not being afraid to gently probe*
  - *Asking 'why'*

Jen Burnham, lead specialist midwife for vulnerable women, Royal Free NHS FT (Barnet Hospital).

Antenatal care

The booking appointment, usually carried out between 8 and 12 weeks' gestation, in the context of PMI, is important to determine pre-existing mental health conditions or to establish risk factors that predispose the woman to develop PMI further into the pregnancy or during the postnatal period. It is the opportunity to begin to build a respectful and trusting relationship between midwife and woman that will continue throughout the antenatal period (and in some cases beyond). Therefore information-gathering in a sensitive and non-judgemental capacity is essential to create a safe environment for the women to disclose information.

It is important for the midwife to be aware of the following risk factors:

- History of mental health problems
- Childhood abuse and neglect
- Domestic violence
- Interpersonal conflict
- Inadequate social support
- Alcohol or drug abuse
- Unplanned or unwanted pregnancy
- Migration status

Previous miscarriage, stillbirth or neonatal death are also more likely to lead to mental health problems in both parents; therefore it is important to take a detailed obstetric history and offer further support if required (PHE, 2019).

Anxiety and depression

Anxiety and depression are common during pregnancy and affect approximately 10–15 out of every 100 pregnant women (RCPsyc, 2018; see

Chapter 1 for further information). Pregnancy is a major life event, which, for most women, brings excitement and trepidation all at once. Therefore it is worth remembering that 'anxiety' itself is a normal human response to both good and bad life events, but for some women, the constant feelings of anxiety can become debilitating and exhausting.

There may be many factors that contribute to women developing anxiety during pregnancy. Women who are vulnerable are most at risk. Some women may have experienced increased anxiety for most of their lives and pregnancy may exacerbate this further. The vulnerabilities which may predispose women to anxiety during pregnancy should be explored by the midwife during every antenatal appointment.

Anxiety relating to pregnancy itself, or *pregnancy-specific anxiety*, has been categorised as a distinct syndrome (Huizink, Mulder, Robles de Medina, Visser, & Buitelaar, 2004). Pregnancy-specific anxiety refers to distinct worries relating to labour and birth, the health of the baby and expected changes in a woman's role (Robertson Blackmore, Gustafsson, Gilchrist, Wyman, & O'Connor, 2016). One prospective cohort study found that pregnancy-specific anxiety was heightened during the third trimester and that nulliparous women reported higher childbirth anxiety than parous mothers (Khalesi & Bokaie, 2018). This is not to be confused with tokophobia, which is a severe, overwhelming fear of pregnancy and childbirth (see Chapter 1).

The Generalised Anxiety Disorder Scale (GAD-2) is a tool used to help identify anxiety in pregnancy. Although this tool is recommended because of its good screening accuracy in the general population, there appears to be a limited evidence base in perinatal populations (Sinesi, Maxwell, O'Carroll, & Cheyne, 2019). Therefore these scales should be used to identify *potential* problems, and if concerns are raised, referral should be made to specialist perinatal teams.

Table 7.1: Example of antenatal screening questions

Whooley questions

- During the past month, have you often been bothered by feeling depressed or hopeless?
- During the past month, have you often been bothered by having little interest or pleasure in doing things?

  (NICE, 2014)

Example of GAD-2 screening tool

- Over the last 2 weeks, how often have you been bothered by feeling nervous, anxious or on-edge?
- Over the last 2 weeks, how often have you been bothered by not being able to stop or control worrying? (NICE, 2014)

Signs that anxiety may be becoming a mental health problem

- feelings of anxiety are very strong and last for a long time
- fears or worries are out of proportion to the situation
- avoiding situations that might cause anxiety
- worries feel very distressing and are hard to control
- regularly experiencing symptoms of anxiety, which may or may not include panic attacks
- finding everyday life difficult and unable to enjoy things (MIND, 2017)

Midwives should enquire about women's emotional wellbeing at every antenatal and postnatal contact, offering support where required. It is important that, on first contact, a thorough history is taken to identify mental health problems, which can be broad and should not be limited to anxiety and depression (Nagle & Farrelly, 2018). Referral to a specialist mental health midwife should be arranged with high-risk women at the first antenatal booking visit (if an issue has been identified at this point) to provide information on early intervention and access to services (Nagle & Farrelly, 2018). Depending on the severity of anxiety, intervention may include access to cognitive behavioural therapy (CBT) (see Chapter 3) and medication when required (NICE, 2014).

Table 7.2: Further guidance on screening for anxiety and depression

If a woman responds positively to either of the anxiety or depression identification tools, the following is recommended:

- If a woman is at risk of developing a mental health problem or there is clinical concern, consider using the Edinburgh Postnatal Depression Scale (EPDS) or the Patient Health Questionnaire (PHQ-9) as part of a full assessment or referring the woman to her general practitioner (GP). If a severe mental health problem is suspected, consider referring the woman to a mental health professional.
- If a woman scores 3 or more on the GAD-2 scale, consider using the GAD-7 scale for further assessment or referring the woman to her GP. If a severe mental health problem is suspected, consider referring her to a mental health professional.
- If a woman scores less than 3 on the GAD-2 scale but you are still concerned she may have an anxiety disorder, ask the following question: *Do you find yourself avoiding places or activities and does this cause you problems?*
- If she responds positively, consider using the GAD-7 scale for further assessment or referring the woman to her GP or, if a severe mental health problem is suspected, to a mental health professional.

(NICE, 2014).

Case Study 7.1   Anxiety and panic attacks during pregnancy

At the booking appointment, Lisa disclosed to her midwife that she had a history of severe anxiety and panic attacks. This was Lisa's first baby; she was 28 years old and smoked approximately 10 cigarettes per day. After the midwife's gentle probing, Lisa revealed that she still suffered from anxiety on a daily basis and that hospitals were a significant trigger for her. She was not taking medication but had received CBT in the past. Lisa was referred to the vulnerable women's team, which provided continuity of care.

As the pregnancy progressed, Lisa's anxiety became worse. After discussion with Lisa, the following plan was put in place:

- Lisa requested to have her baby in the co-located birth centre.
- A tour of the birth centre was arranged for Lisa and her partner.
- Antenatal appointments were to take place in the hospital so that Lisa could become familiar with the hospital environment, including the birth centre.
- Lisa was scheduled to meet other members of the vulnerable women's team who might be on-call for intrapartum care. This was to help Lisa become familiar with the midwife who might look after her during labour.

At 36 weeks, Lisa's growth scan revealed that the baby's growth had reduced. Lisa was advised to have two weekly CTGs. She became more anxious about the health of her baby and extremely worried that she would not be able to give birth in the birth centre. Thankfully, at her next scan, the baby's growth had increased. However, her panic attacks had become more frequent recently. She was able to use distraction techniques as a coping mechanism. The techniques included the following:

- Drinking a glass of cold water
- Cooling down with a fan
- Playing games on her phone or tablet

A new plan was put in place for Lisa:

- To have a CTG on the labour ward when admitted in labour. If CTG was normal, care was to be continued on the birth centre.
- Take a tour of the labour ward and birthing room.
- Discuss what might happen if labour becomes high-risk.
- If Lisa had a panic attack during labour, use distraction techniques, usually games on her phone, if possible.

Lisa gave birth to a baby boy 1 week later on the labour ward with no complications. During the postnatal period she became anxious when she found it difficult to breastfeed and chose to bottle-feed instead. She was worried that she was not doing the best thing for her baby. The midwives supported her and did not pressure her to breastfeed. Lisa was discharged to the health visitor 28 days later. Her mood was stable, and she was enjoying motherhood.

Part 2: Intrapartum care

The labour experience is often a frightening time for women. For nulliparous women or those who have experienced a traumatic birth, the uncertainty of what to expect during the labour process can be daunting, confusing and stressful. However, it is worth considering the following three fundamental aspects of psychological care for women who are in labour.

- Expectation
- Control
- Outcome

Expectation

Some women have a very clear idea of what they would like to happen during labour and birth. This is usually documented in the form of a birth plan discussion which can be used to facilitate the provision of holistic, individualised care (Jackson, Anderson, & Marshall, 2020). For women with mental health issues and complex needs, a more detailed birth plan may be required. The birth plan is the very essence of women-centred care and it is important to ensure that the women's voice is not lost during the often challenging time of labour and birth. Ideally, vulnerable women who are under the care of a team specialising in mental health and complex needs will be under the continuity of carer model; however, this may not always be the case. Therefore it is important that all midwives who provide intrapartum care have a good understanding of how to support women with mental health issues or complex emotional needs.

Communication is crucial to helping the woman achieve her objectives and providing effective, safe and supportive care during labour (NHS England, 2016; RCOG, 2016). A recent study investigated care during pregnancy and reported outcomes in women with mental health problems. A significant finding from this study was that women with PMI reported health care professionals less likely to speak to them in a way they could understand, did not listen to them and did not respect them as individuals (Henderson, Jomeen, & Redshaw, 2018). It was also found that women with PMI were significantly more worried about labour and birth and were less satisfied with their experience of birth, finding it more stressful compared with women without mental health problems (Henderson et al., 2018). The reasons women were dissatisfied included being left alone at a time that worried them, poor interactions with staff and less confidence and trust in staff (Henderson et al., 2018). Interestingly, women with PMI reported their labour and birth to have gone better than expected (Henderson et al., 2018). In some ways, this is unsurprising considering that women with PMI may have higher levels of anxiety surrounding labour and birth.

Effective communication is central to creating a safe, psychological environment for the woman and her partner. Thinking about the words we use, the way we say them and the tone or our voice are important factors in communication because of how the woman might perceive them. In the words of Mavis Kirkham, good communication is 'the vehicle by which all else is learnt and relationships are built' (Kirkham, 1993).

For women who have experienced trauma due to sexual abuse or previous obstetric and traumatic birth experiences, the use of a particular word, phrases and colloquialisms could be harmful. As a general rule, the use of language that infantilises, disempowers or condescends to women in labour should be avoided. Indeed this can prove harmful if women are subjected to phrases such as 'good girl' or being told just 'to lie back' as these can retraumatise and cause an enactment of abuse. Many women do not disclose sexual abuse, yet this could be at the root of existing mental health issues; therefore in all labours, midwives should take this into account (Montgomery, Pope, & Rogers, 2015).

Practice learning point for effective communication for women with PMI during labour

- *Speak calmly and with kindness.*
- *Communicate all aspects of clinical care in a way the woman and her partner can understand.*
- *Speak clearly and with clarity.*
- *Actively listen.*
- *Validate the woman's feelings.*
- *Ask, 'What can I do for you?'*
- *Find out what the women's coping mechanisms are and work with the woman to support her.*
- *When discussing the woman's care with the multi-disciplinary team, remember to include the woman and her partner.*
- *Consider the language being used in labour. Could words, phrases or tone be described as disempowering or cause the woman to feel infantilised?*
- *If you have to leave the room at any time, ask the woman if it is an appropriate time to do so, and explain what you are doing.*
- *Sometimes the woman might want some time alone with her partner during labour; if it is safe to do so, ask if she would like this.*

Control

It is widely accepted that factors facilitating a positive birth experience include having a sense of control during birth (Czarnocka & Slade, 2000; Ozlo et al., 2018), an opportunity for active involvement in care (Jackson et al., 2020; NHS England, 2016; Ozlo et al., 2018; RCOG, 2016) and supportive and responsive care (Ozlo et al., 2018). A sense of control is important in both an internal and an external sense, internally as a psychological coping mechanism and externally as an active participant in one's own care. Internal control may include a sense of self-control, such as thoughts, behaviours and coping with the pain of labour (Ozlo et al., 2018), while external control is described as the woman's involvement in her care, understanding what is happening during the birth process and participating in decisions about her care (Ford & Ayers, 2008; Green & Baston, 2003; Ozlo et al., 2018).

Creating a safe birth space in midwifery led units and at home

Working with the woman to create a safe birthplace is important in helping her maintain a sense of control over her birth. As clinicians, when considering a 'safe' birth space in relation to place of birth, focus is often placed on assessment of physical suitability, evaluating the obstetric and medical factors which may influence a recommendation or discussion around planned home or hospital birth. Indeed, NICE (2017) provides discussions around place of birth options for nulliparous and multiparous women based on documented risk factors.

In relation to decision making for women with perinatal mental health issues, NICE guidance suggests that specific recommendations for place of birth are only specified for women experiencing a psychiatric disorder requiring current inpatient care ('*indicating increased risk suggesting planned birth at obstetric unit*') and those under current outpatient psychiatric care ('*indicating individual assessment when planning place of birth*') (NICE, 2014).

The implication is that, for many women who present for maternity care in the presence of perinatal mental ill health, physical or psychological trauma and phobia, consideration of birthing anywhere outside of a hospital may be something that had not crossed their minds despite this being a viable and potentially beneficial option. This phenomenon is not unusual, with many studies identifying that women are often unaware that they have a choice of birthplace and assume that a hospital birth is the only option (Hollowell, Li, Malouf, & Buchanan, 2016). In the absence, therefore, of defined medical or obstetric conditions and those identified within the NICE (2017) guidelines, there is no evidence that women should not be offered a choice in place of birth. Unless the risks of birthing at home are such that there is an increased chance of exacerbation of a woman's condition, where birth in an obstetric unit would be preferable to reduce that risk, birth in a midwifery led unit (MLU) or at home should be an option presented to that woman when planning her care. It is acknowledged that birth outside of a hospital will not be the right choice for everyone; however, perinatal mental ill health, trauma and phobia should not preclude birth at home or in an MLU due to maternal or caregivers' unfamiliarity with the concept and ill placed concerns around homebirth or birth in an MLU.

The following addresses issues and considerations for women who remain suitable for homebirth and MLU but happen to have perinatal mental health issues. For the purposes of birthplace and planning for intrapartum care discussions, reference to the inter- and multi-disciplinary team refers to (but is not limited to):

- The midwife or midwives providing continuity or intrapartum care
- Obstetricians
- Consultant midwives
- Neonatologists/paediatricians
- The GP
- Perinatal mental health teams
- Psychiatrist and psychiatric team
- Community psychiatric nurses
- Social workers
- Pharmacists

The evidence for homebirth and birth in midwifery led units

The evidence for the safety of homebirth for women who have low obstetric and medical risk has been well established, and in the case of low-risk multiparous women, it may be safer than birth in an obstetric led unit. This is primarily because rates of intervention are reduced and normal birth rate increased (Brocklehurst et al., 2011; Hutton, Reitsma, & Kaufman, 2009; Kennare, Keirse, Tucker, & Chan, 2010; Zielinski, Ackerson, & Low, 2015) as well as an acknowledgment of the benefits of outside of hospital and midwife-led care likely result in a higher chance of spontaneous vaginal birth (NHS England, 2016; Sandall, Soltani, Gates, Shennan, & Devane, 2016).

This is in direct opposition to the standardisation of maternity care, which by its very nature removes the individual from the process and therefore any means of adapting to individual circumstances, which may hinder the progress of birth. The National Maternity Review: Better Births (NHS England, 2016) acknowledges this and has set the standard for improving individualised care and continuity of care, which is being realised throughout the establishment and across the UK in continuity of care teams, including dedicated homebirth teams and case loading midwives.

Risk discourse

Risk perception is extremely personal in nature and highly subjective (Lee, Ayers, & Holden, 2016); therefore it is vital that any advice given is done so in a manner that is balanced, based on individual circumstance and unbiased. Studies have shown that factors influencing women's choices relating to birthplace are multifaceted and relate to previous birth experiences; information gained from families, friends, midwives and other clinicians; personal preference and experiences of health care services and, importantly, the views of multi-disciplinary team members and their perception of risk, which are often at odds with the perception of the woman (Coxon, Sandall, & Fulop, 2014; Coxon, Chisholm, Malouf, Rowe, & Hollowell, 2017; Healy, Humphreys, & Kennedy, 2016, 2017). When physiological birth is viewed through the lens of risk, there is transference from support of the physiological process to risk management, which can have a negative impact on the nature of supporting true informed choice (Healy et al., 2017; Naylor Smith et al., 2018).

The NMC (2018) Code is clear in its assertions that midwives should support women's informed choices, regardless of whether the clinician agrees with that choice, and indeed it is also clear that the information provided should be evidence-based in nature. This is of acute importance where women make choices which, by whatever mechanism, appear to be 'against guideline' or 'against medical advice'. The nature of a woman's complexity or vulnerability must therefore be fairly weighed against the best-known evidence and balanced information and advice, presenting the risks and benefits from a non-biased perspective, and presented to the woman to allow her to reach a decision regarding her care (NICE, 2014). In discussing risk, the ruling in Montgomery v. Lanarkshire Health Board (2015) ensures that health care providers must enter into a dialogue that is sensitive to the individual's needs and situation, informing her of her options (including the right to decline care) as well as an appreciation of human rights legislation that protects a woman's right to choose her place of birth (WHO, 2012).

The right to choose and to decline care or medical advice

It is worth noting at this juncture that even in the presence of a recommendation of birthplace, a woman cannot be required to comply. Unless there are concerns around mental capacity to make decisions, a woman's choices cannot be overridden nor coercion applied as this would be unethical and unlawful. Choice is and continues to be a fundamental principle of modern maternity care (DOH, 2007).

It is therefore of utmost importance to work with women to facilitate their choices in the presence of information individual to their needs. NICE (2017) explicitly illustrates medical and obstetric conditions indicating increased risk. Thus birth being recommended in an obstetric unit, however outside of these recommendations, should involve individual risk assessment, particularly where these recommendations are made due to the following:

+ Anxiety
+ Depression
+ Previous trauma
+ Phobia
+ Personality disorder
+ Previous sexual abuse

Whilst it is acknowledged that ongoing treatment and care plans for mental health issues may have implications regarding place of birth, they should not preclude discussion of choice, indeed where a woman chooses to birth at home or in an MLU against the recommendation of the inter- or multi-disciplinary team. It is imperative that respectful and caring discourse be entered into with a goal of coming to a mutual agreement or compromise as to how an individualised plan might be reached. NICE (2017) also requires a culture of respectful care, including behaviours and communication with the woman in relation to her choices, regardless of whether her ultimate decisions align with what we as health care professionals might ourselves choose.

When facilitating discussion and informed decision making, we must reflect on whether the presence of mental ill health, physical or psychological trauma and phobia should be an influencing factor in choice of birthplace, from the perspective of obstetric and medical factors, and how homebirth may be considered to have a protective factor.

Benefits of homebirth for women with perinatal mental health issues

Continuity of care

Studies have shown that continuity of care (CoC) should remain one of the cornerstones of midwifery practice, improving provision of a unified care journey for the woman and her family and outcomes such as maternal satisfaction and rates of physiological birth. The continuity model has been shown to be effective in all areas of care and fundamentally in those with challenging psychosocial and mental health complexity (Brocklehurst et al., 2011; Hodnett et al., 2008; Rayment-Jones, Murrells, & Sandall, 2015; Renfrew et al., 2014; Sandall et al., 2016).

For women who choose to homebirth or MLUs in the presence of psychological factors, the CoC model is ideally placed to provide support and improve outcomes, with the inter- and multi-disciplinary team featuring within that model and coordinated by the primary named midwife. NICE (2014) acknowledges that some mental health conditions, including a range of anxiety and depressive disorders, are under-recognised within the context of pregnancy. Therefore CoC allows for initial assessment of required support, ongoing familiarity with the condition and monitoring of symptoms and appropriate referrals, as well as building a trusting relationship to facilitate disclosure of difficulties and co-created pathways of care. For women with more serious diagnoses and established care plans, the benefits of CoC are therefore obvious.

Autonomy, control and birth environment

It is widely acknowledged that a clinical birth environment can hinder the physiological processes required to birth safely and confidently. Bright lights, loud alarms and beeps, clinical smells, uniformed clinical staff who are unfamiliar and hospital routine can all have a detrimental effect in disturbing birth and subsequent outcomes.

Birth environment is a fundamental consideration for women's intrapartum experiences, consequent wellbeing and, for women with perinatal mental ill health, trauma or phobia. This may influence perceptions of control, which, alongside provision of adequate and appropriately conveyed and understood information, is necessary for positive psychological outcome in relation to birth (Green, Coupland, & Kitzinger, 1990). This is acknowledged by NICE (2017), recognising that, for any woman, pregnancy and birth are life experiences which can be emotionally significant and intense. Therefore, to ensure that the woman remains in control, she and her family should be listened to with compassion.

Where birth is facilitated in clinical, institution-based environments, influenced by routine and the medical model of care, women can experience feelings of distress, disempowerment, loss of control and heightened vulnerability (Green et al., 1990), all of which could reasonably be expected to have a detrimental effect and exacerbate

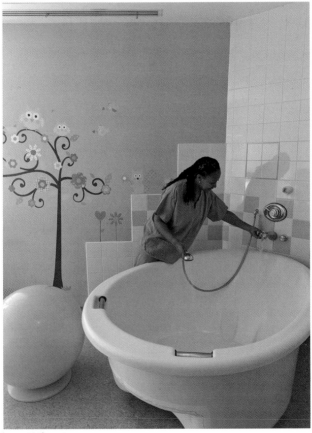

Fig 7.3 **Birth centre room.**

mental ill health or previous trauma. Conversely, it can be hypothesised that birth facilitated in a home or home-like environment could have an empowering effect on women, influencing improved obstetric and psychological outcomes. A Cochrane review undertaken by Hodnett et al. (2010) found that women who had active involvement in their decision making had a more positive birth experience and outcomes from a physical, psychological and emotional perspective. Additionally, where birth is conducted in a non-delivery suite environment or one in which modifications have been made to mimic out-of-hospital care, women needed less analgesia, augmentation, intervention and operative birth and had a greater perception of support of caregivers and security. These findings have been reflected in Lock and Gibb (2003) study, which explored the power of birthplace and the Birthplace Study (Brocklehurst et al., 2011).

Familiarity of surroundings and caregivers, physiology of birth

In order for birth to progress in such a way as to remain unhindered physiologically, many factors must be supported and protected. The familiar oxytocin feedback loop will progress when the labouring woman feels safe, undisturbed and supported, allowing her to respond to the natural and unconscious signals her body sends – swaying, moving, vocalising. For this to happen, the woman must hand over her body to the involuntary impulses and let go of control, self-awareness and external arousal, which could overwhelm the hypothalamus-directed birth process.

To support these processes, it is important to establish general principles of a labour environment that is supportive and aids the support of physiological processes, none of which will be unfamiliar to midwives, for example:

- Low lighting
- Aromatherapy or familiar and comforting smells
- Quiet and calm environment
- Comfortable temperature, under the woman's control
- Removal of clinical equipment from the eyeline
- Privacy, not being overheard
- Maintaining dignity
- Nutrition and hydration of choice
- Not being openly observed
- Control over who is in the room with them
- Gentle encouragement to mobilise

Specific considerations for women with perinatal mental health issues choosing MLU/homebirth

To a large extent, the nature and management of the woman's presenting condition will determine any challenges that might require discussion and planning for a homebirth. On the whole, women who are suffering from less serious mental health issues in the absence of other medical or obstetric risk factors/considered 'low risk', may require only monitoring and support as per NICE guidelines and local trust policies, the place of birth only being incidental to their care plan. The following, however, may need further consideration.

Birth preferences and planning

Listen to the woman and facilitate open and frank discussion around her preferences for birth including the provision of appropriate information (Hinton, Dumelow, Rowe, & Hollowell, 2018). In the first instance it may be useful to understand why the woman has opted for homebirth or MLU. In some cases it can be simply the recognition of the benefits of homebirth or MLU care. However, it may be due to a phobia or difficult experience in a previous pregnancy unrelated to a current or previous mental health issue or related to trauma sustained in a previous pregnancy (i.e. stillbirth or birth mode) (Gribbin, 2017). Careful consideration of issues such as agoraphobia and other conditions which may lead to difficulty in transfer (see section titled 'Transfer') or the offering of particular interventions in an emergency such as vaginal examinations should be carefully and sensitively explored alongside frank but sensitive discussions of how these may be managed should the need arise.

The motivations for choosing homebirth or MLU are very personal; therefore it is imperative that as primary caregivers we understand these motivations and build these into the birth preferences, taking into account the 'what ifs'. Explore the woman's choices and preferences and develop a birth preference strategy for labour. Consider communication, examinations, specific interventions, transfer, pain relief and postnatal considerations. The key is to ensure that control is not removed from the woman and to encourage those strategies to be flexible in the event of the preferences needing to adapt or change to the situation.

Conversely, women may find interventions, such as hypnobirthing and other techniques using visualisation and affirmations, useful in managing anxiety which often replace words such as 'contraction' or 'pain with 'surges' and 'pressure' or 'sensation'. It is important to understand that when women have engaged and invested in these descriptors, they are respected and that every effort is made to reflect these wishes in the language used.

Supporting the woman and her choice

- *Sensitively approach discussions around motivations for choosing or declining recommendations for a particular place of birth.*
- *Consider offering networking opportunities for the woman with other women and families who have experienced particular places of birth, perhaps at group meet ups/meet the midwives.*
- *Develop a template for exploring birth preferences as a means of co-creating agreed pathways of care.*
- *Consider individualised tours of clinical areas such as delivery suites, wards and neonatal units in conjunction with the inter- and multi-disciplinary team to develop familiarity.*
- *Ensure early and appropriate referral for further support following disclosure of difficulties (i.e. counselling and GP).*

Medication

Women who are on regular medications to treat mental ill health will have regular reviews and treatment adjusted according to the pregnancy and in discussion with their obstetric consultant and mental health team. Many medications, if taken through pregnancy, do not influence midwifery and intrapartum care. Some medications, however, will require that continuous fetal health monitoring is required in labour or that the neonate is monitored or reviewed post birth for withdrawal. This will need to be considered alongside the inter- and multi-disciplinary teams' care plan, co-created with the woman, as this will influence recommendations for birthplace.

Medication

- *Ensure early and ongoing referral for medication review where necessary.*
- *Instigate discussions early regarding medication regimes that need to recommence or be reviewed immediately post birth.*
- *Involve the neonatal team in discussions surrounding birth plans if medication continues through pregnancy.*
- *Always include medication regimes in antenatal discussions around immediate and ongoing care needs.*
- *If medication regime is to recommence postnatally, try to ensure that medication is available at home.*

Transfer

Depending on the clinical situation, transfer from homebirth or MLU can occur for a number of factors such as intrapartum for analgesia, concerns of progress, obstetric or neonatal emergency or monitoring post birth. The Birthplace Study (2011) showed that for low-risk nulliparous women, the transfer rate for planned homebirths was 45%, 35% for freestanding midwifery units and 40% for planned alongside midwifery units. For low-risk multiparous women, these figures fall to 12% for planned homebirths, 9% for freestanding midwifery unit births and 13% for alongside midwifery units. Care and time should be taken in discussing these eventualities alongside discussion of how this might be managed, for example, by ambulance from homebirth or freestanding MLU or through clinical areas which may have been involved in previous traumatic experiences. In some cases, a plan may have been made with neonatal and obstetric teams that a review or observations on the neonate, as a result of maternal antenatal mental health medication, is appropriate. If this is the case, the pathway should be clear and documented in the birth plan with the woman, her family and the multi-disciplinary team.

| Practice learning point |

Safe plan for transfer
- *Discuss and reflect with the woman as many eventualities as possible and the potential pathways for care.*
- *Consider a visit to potentially problematic clinical areas during the antenatal period in consultation with the mental health team to explore feelings and reactions to that area.*
- *Ensure that, where possible, the same caregiver remains throughout and after transfer or handover to a continuity team.*
- *Where there are pre-existing plans for postnatal transfer for review or observations, ensure that every multi-disciplinary team member is aware and has access to the written plan of care.*

Strategies for building relationships between the MDT (perinatal psychiatric and nursing colleagues) and support for midwives facilitating birth at home for women with complex health needs

Adjustments and considerations for supporting women with mental health issues in their birthplace choices are centred around co-created birth pre-planning, communication, respectful care and an understanding of the woman's particular condition. By far, one of the most important considerations is an effective inter- and multi-disciplinary team working towards the same goal of women-centred care. By definition, this should mean that they are involved in all aspects of care planning.

Whilst homebirth and MLU care are traditionally seen as the domain of the midwife, the duty to work cooperatively within the multi-disciplinary team still exists. Where a woman has chosen to birth in these environments in the presence of current or previous perinatal mental ill health or other conditions, it is imperative that care continues within that team, providing support and developing relationships that are trusting and comfortable. Madeley, Williams, and McNiven (2019) studied the experiences of midwives providing such care and showed that the most successful teams functioned well when the wider multi-disciplinary team was involved early and worked within a woman-centred approach. Consultant midwives were considered fundamental in the planning and advocacy of women in these situations, particularly where there existed any dissonance between individual disciplines, bridging midwifery advocacy and the team as well as allowing time to explore issues and develop birth preferences with the woman through birth choice clinics and birth preparation.

Practice learning point

Facilitating choice of place of birth

- *Where possible, instigate discussions early in pregnancy to explore a woman's understanding of her choices in relation to birthplace and expectations in this pregnancy.*
- *Develop and embed guidelines and standard operating procedures, particularly for care pathways where care might be considered 'outside of guidelines'.*
- *Ensure all communication between and within the inter- and multi-disciplinary team includes the woman and that it is clear, open and undertaken in a timely manner to facilitate discussion.*
- *Develop a relationship with psychiatric and mental health services and explore their understanding of birthplace choices and provide information supporting their own knowledge of birthplace choice.*
- *Ensure that the multi-disciplinary team, including obstetricians, psychiatrists, nurses and the mental health team, is provided with information and education around maternal choices and evidence supporting homebirth and MLU care.*
- *Where possible, ensure continuity of maternity care and care provider, preferably a named midwife, obstetrician and consultant midwife alongside the mental health team/services.*
- *Acknowledging that all clinicians are responsible for their clinical actions and omissions (as well as acting within their own scope of practice and competence sphere), ensure that mechanisms are in place to develop their own skills, and document and reflect on episodes of care for the ongoing improvement of services.*

Practice learning point

How can the midwife help to facilitate the woman's sense of control during intrapartum care?

- *Discuss the woman's birth plan and preferred place of birth with her at an appropriate point during intrapartum care, ideally when the woman is first admitted onto the labour ward or the birth centre or when the midwife arrives at the women's home.*
- *Ensure that the multi-disciplinary team members are aware of the women's birth plan.*
- *Work with the woman during labour to ensure her wants and needs are met, including pain relief strategies, positions for labour and any other request the woman might put forward.*
- *Ensure effective communication throughout intrapartum care.*
- *If complications arise during labour, facilitate discussions with the women using evidence-based guidance and ensure she is supported in her choices.*
- *In the event of an emergency, try, time of urgency permitting, to explain to the woman and her partner what is happening. It is important that after the emergency scenario, a full debrief is had with the woman and her partner and staff involved.*

Outcome-postpartum

The outcome of birth and the impact it has will be different for all women and their families. What might be considered a positive birth experience for one woman might be considered negative by the next. Birth experience and what it means is subjective, unique to every woman, including the physiological mechanism of the birth process and the psychological journey a woman takes throughout pregnancy and into motherhood.

Even if, by clinical standards, the birth appears to have gone well, the woman may have a very different perception of events. In fact, up to one-third of mothers rate their childbirth as traumatic (Sandoz et al., 2019), and women with mental health conditions are more likely to experience birth as a traumatic event (Simpson & Catling, 2016). A small minority of women who experience a traumatic birth may develop posttraumatic stress disorder (PTSD) as discussed in Chapter 1 (Graaf, Honig, Pampus, & Stramrood, 2018). Factors that appear to contribute to a traumatic birth experience include a lack or loss of control, sub-optimal communication with health practitioners and a lack of practical and emotional support during labour (Graaf et al., 2018).

The combination of supporting expectation and helping to facilitate the women's sense of control in the birth environment may offer some protective factors against psychological birth trauma. However, birth is unpredictable and events may stray from the woman's anticipated birth plan, causing distress to the woman and her partner. Up to 16% of women who have experienced a traumatic scenario during labour, such as an emergency caesarean section or preterm birth, develop PTSD (Furuta et al., 2018).

There is some suggestion that asking postpartum women about their birth experience and how their thoughts and feelings connect with it may be helpful in identifying women at risk of birth trauma and subsequent PTSD (Graaf et al., 2018). Some women have reported that they were not offered support after a traumatic birth and that their thoughts and feelings were not taken seriously (RCOG, 2017). It is recommended by the RCOG that any woman who identifies with having a traumatic birth should be seen and assessed by a perinatal mental health lead who can carry out assessments post childbirth (RCOG, 2017). Information should be given to women on where to seek help should perinatal mental health symptoms develop (RCOG, 2017). This support should also be available for partners.

The development of postpartum mental health conditions appears to be dependent on a number of complex interactions, such as psychological, social and biological, plus environmental and genetic factors (Meltzer-Brody et al., 2018). Four well-established risk factors have been identified in the development of postnatal depression: (1) personal psychiatric history, (2) coincidental adverse life events, (3) poor quality of relationship with intimate partner and (4) insufficient social support (Rowe & Fisher, 2010). Although a traumatic birth experience may contribute to the development of mental health conditions postpartum, the evidence for this is less reliable (Rowe & Fisher, 2010).

It is also important to take into account the woman's home environment and the mental health of her partner (see further discussion in Chapter 6). The RCOG Maternal Mental Health-Women's Voices Report (2017) found that 12% of women (one in eight) who responded to the survey conducted by the RCOG to explore perinatal mental health said that their partner had experienced mental health issues. The following issues were identified from the survey in relation to a partner's mental health:

- Health care professionals focused on the health of mother and baby and seldom on the health of the partner.
- Health care professionals failed to ask about the mental health of partners.

- Women reported that their partners, especially men, were less likely to seek help proactively.
- In some cases, support for traumatic events, such as recurrent miscarriages or traumatic birth, was offered to the mother and not the father.
- A number of women felt that their partner's mental health put a strain on their relationship and how they were able to support each other. In some cases, this led to a relationship breakdown (RCOG, 2017).

Infant feeding

Infant feeding is another factor that can cause women stress and anxiety during the postnatal period. It is not unusual for midwives to witness tired, stressed women blaming themselves for finding it difficult to breastfeed. Some women may feel pressured to breastfeed and, if they choose not to, may feel judged, adding to further stress (Chaput et al., 2016; RCOG, 2017).

The link between breastfeeding difficulties and postpartum depression (PPD) is well documented (Brown, Rance, & Bennett, 2015; Chaput et al., 2016). PPD appears to be associated with short breastfeeding duration and multiple reasons for stopping (Brown et al., 2015). PPD was especially associated with women deciding to stop breastfeeding due to pain and physical issues with breastfeeding (Brown et al., 2015).

A protective factor against PPD appears to be women receiving good infant feeding support (Chaput et al., 2016). Help with breastfeeding and supporting women's choices if they decide not to breastfeed is also important to ensure maternal mental health during the postpartum period (RCOG, 2017). It is important that the midwife discuss signs of PPD with the woman and her family and that the woman is able to distinguish between 'normal' baby blues and actual PPD.

Breastfeeding tips to support women with perinatal mental illness

- During pregnancy, at around 28 weeks' gestation, all mothers must be given the opportunity to have a 'meaningful antenatal conversation' around caring and feeding her baby by her midwife, whether face to face or by phone/virtual platform. This will include the offer of a discussion/information around the health benefits of breastfeeding for both mother and baby and the reassurance of support she will receive in hospital. It should also include signposting to support in her local community plus national breastfeeding helplines. This will ensure that mothers-to-be feel prepared and well supported in their choice of feeding.

- Mothers who have a history of or are currently being treated for depression, anxiety or any form of mental illness will need support, reassurance and clear information around any concerns they may have regarding medication and breastfeeding. The Breastfeeding Network UK is an evidence-based source of information which professionals can signpost women to alongside medical support from her GP and chosen maternity unit.

- Involving her birth partner, friend or family member helps her feel supported by the most important people in her life; this begins in pregnancy and especially relates to the importance of antenatal classes where birth partners are encouraged to attend.

- As professionals we must respect and acknowledge how a woman chooses to feed her baby by giving her evidence-based support around building a happy and loving relationship with her baby. A woman should never feel pressured to breastfeed or feel guilty about bottle feeding. She needs to feel supported.

- After the birth of her baby, mothers must be supported with skin-to-skin contact unless clinically contra-indicated. Skin-to-skin contact enhances bonding and attachment and also initiates the first breastfeed. If a mother chooses to bottle feed, skin-to-skin should still be encouraged, as it is for all mothers and babies. Midwives should enable a mother to enjoy the closeness, bonding and skin contact for as long as she wishes.

- Keeping mothers and babies together facilitates early attachment and supports the mother's mental wellbeing as well as the baby's short- and long-term health including brain development. If, for whatever reason, a mother is unable to see her baby, supporting parents by way of virtual platforms such as V Create (Neonatal Units) should be facilitated. This enables mother and partner to see and hear their baby. Muslin cloths that have been close to both mother and baby can be used so both can smell the scent of each other and provide support with lactation. All of this will raise levels of oxytocin, resulting in strengthening the mother–baby dyad, brain development, relaxation and loving feelings.

Jenny Whelehan, infant feeding specialist midwife, Royal Free Hospital

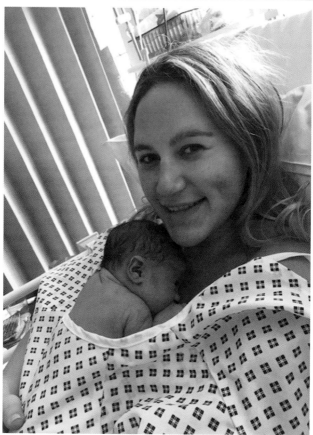

Fig 7.4 Breastfeeding mother.

Conclusion

PMI is vast and it is advised that this chapter should be supported with further reading, especially texts that document women's lived experiences of PMI. Every woman is individual, as is every woman's experience of pregnancy, and widening our scope of practice to embrace PMI is crucial to offer women holistic care. Opening our eyes and ears, reading between the lines and softly teasing out unspoken cues that might indicate hidden trauma, pain or anxiety is essential if we are to identify women requiring mental health intervention. We might never be able to fully understand another person's perception of the world, the content of their thoughts or the emotional context of their life, but with a little understanding, empathy and patience, we can at least offer a hand to hold on to.

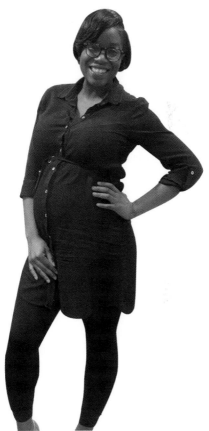

Fig 7.5 Pregnant woman.

POINTS FOR REFLECTION

- How might you ensure that a safe space is created for the woman to disclose any mental health concerns to you during antenatal and postnatal care?
- You have been asked to care for a woman with known PMI during labour. What would you do to ensure that both her psychological and her physical needs are met?
- How might you ensure that you offer the full range of choice regarding place of birth for women with PMI?

References

Birthplace Study (BMJ) (2011). *Perinatal and maternal outcomes by planned place of birth for healthy women with low risk pregnancies: the Birthplace in England national prospective cohort study*. https://doi.org/10.1136/bmj.d7400.

Brocklehurst, P., Hardy, P., Hollowell, J., Linsell, L., Macfarlane, A., McCourt, C., … , Petrou, S., et al. (2011). Perinatal and maternal outcomes by planned place of birth for healthy women with low risk pregnancies: The birthplace in England national prospective cohort study. *BMJ*, *343*, d7400.

Brown, A., Rance, J., & Bennett, P. (2015). Understanding the relationship between breastfeeding and postnatal depression: The role of pain and physical difficulties: *Journal of Advanced Nursing*. https://onlinelibrary.wiley.com/doi/full/10.1111/jan.12832.

Chaput, K. H., Nettle-Aguirre, A., Stat, P., Musto, R., Adair, C. E., & Tough, S. (2016). Breastfeeding difficulties and supports and risk of postpartum depression in a cohort of women who have given birth in Calgary: A prospective cohort study. *Cmaj Open*. http://cmajopen.ca/content/4/1/E103.abstract?maxtoshow=&HITS=10&hits=10&RESULTFORMAT=&andorexacttitle=and&andorexacttitleabs=and&fulltext=breastfeed%252C+breastfeeding%252C+%2522breast+feed%2522%252C+%2522Baby+Friendly%2522%252C+breastmilk&andorexactfulltext=or&searchid=1&FIRSTINDEX=0&fdate=//&resourcetype=HWCIT.

Coates, D., & Foureur, N. (2019). The role and competence of midwives in supporting women with mental health concerns during the perinatal period: A scoping review. *Wiley Online Library*. https://doi.org/10.1111/hsc.12740.

Coxon, K., Chisholm, A., Malouf, R., Rowe, R., & Hollowell, J. (2017). What influences birthplace preferences, choices and decision-making amongst healthy women with straightforward pregnancies in the UK? A qualitative evidence synthesis using a 'best fit' framework approach. *BMC Pregnancy and Childbirth*, *17*(1), 103.

Coxon, K., Sandall, J., & Fulop, N. J. (2014). To what extent are women free to choose where to give birth? How discourses of risk, blame and responsibility influence birthplace decisions. *Health, Risk and Society*, 16(1), 51–67.

Czarnocka, J., & Slade, P. (2000). Prevalence and predictors of post-traumatic stress symptoms following childbirth. *British Journal of Clinical Psychology*, 39(1), 35–51.

Department of Health (DOH). (2007). *Maternity matters: Choice, access and continuity of care in a safe service*. London: Crown.

Doherty, A. M., Crudden, G., Jabbar, F., Sheehan, J. D., & Casey, P. (2019). Suicidality in women with adjustment disorder and depressive episodes attending an Irish perinatal mental health service. *International Journal of Environmental Research & Public Health*. https://www.mdpi.com/1660-4601/16/20/3970/htm.

Ford, E., & Ayers, S. (2008). Stressful events and support during birth: The effect on anxiety, mood and perceived control. *Journal of Anxiety Disorders*. https://pubmed.ncbi.nlm.nih.gov/18789646/.

Furuta, M., Horsch, A., Ng, E. S. W., Bick, D., Spain, D., & Sin, J. (2018). Effectiveness of trauma-focused psychological therapies for treating post-traumatic stress disorder symptoms in women following childbirth: A systematic review and meta-analysis. *Frontiers in Psychiatry*. https://www.ncbi.nlm.nih.gov/pmc/articles/PMC6255986/.

Graaf, L. F., Honig, A., Pampus, M. G., & Stramrood, C. A. I. (2018). Preventing post-traumatic stress disorder following childbirth and traumatic birth experiences: A systematic review. *AOGS*. https://obgyn.onlinelibrary.wiley.com/doi/full/10.1111/aogs.13291.

Green, J., & Baston, H. (2003). Feeling in control during labor: Concepts, correlates, and consequences. *Birth*. https://pubmed.ncbi.nlm.nih.gov/14992154/.

Green, J. M., Coupland, V. A., & Kitzinger, S. (1990). Expectations, experiences and psychological outcomes of childbirth: A prospective study of 825 women. *Birth*, 17(1), 15–24.

Gribbin. C. (2017). Fear of childbirth: The impact of tocophobia (including post-traumatic stress disorder) on normal birth. In K. Jackson & H. Wightman (Eds.), *Normalising challenging or complex childbirth* (pp. 65–81). London: McGraw Hill Education.

Grigoriasdis, S., Wilton, A. S., Kurdyak, P. A., Rhodes, A. E., VonderPorten, E. H., Levitt, A., … Vigood, S. N. (2017). Perinatal suicide in Ontario, Canada: A 15 year population-based study. *CMAJ*. https://www.ncbi.nlm.nih.gov/pmc/articles/PMC5573543/.

Healy, S., Humphreys, E., & Kennedy, C. (2016). Midwives' and obstetricians' perceptions of risk and its impact on clinical practice and decision-making in labour: An integrative review. *Women Birth*, 29(2), 107–116. https://doi.org/10.1016/j.wombi.2015.08.010.

Healy, S., Humphreys, E., & Kennedy, C. (2017). A qualitative exploration of how midwives' and obstetricians' perception of risk affects care practices for low-risk women and normal birth. *Women Birth*, 30(5), 367–375. https://doi.org/10.1016/j.wombi.2017.02.005.

Henderson, J., Jomeen, J., & Redshaw, M. (2018). Care and self-reported outcomes of care experienced by women with mental health problems in pregnancy: Findings from a national survey. *Midwifery*, 56, 171–178.

Hinton, L., Dumelow, C., Rowe, R., & Hollowell, J. (2018). Birthplace choices: What are the information needs of women when choosing where to give birth in England? A qualitative study using online and face to face focus groups. *BMC Pregnancy & Childbirth*, 18(1), 12. https://doi.org/10.1186/s12884-017-1601-4.

Hodnett, E., Downe, S., Edwards, N., et al. (2010). Alternative versus conventional institutional settings for birth. In *Cochrane Database of Systematic Reviews*. Chichester: John Wiley & Sons.

Hodnett, E. D., Hatem, M., Sandall, J., et al. (2008). Continuity of caregivers for care during pregnancy and childbirth. In *Cochrane Database of Systematic Reviews*. Chichester: John Wiley & Sons.

Hollowell, J., Li, Y., Malouf, R., & Buchanan, J. (2016). Women's birthplace preferences in the United Kingdom: A systematic review and narrative synthesis of the quantitative literature. *BMC Pregnancy and Childbirth*, 16(1), 213. https://doi.org/10.1186/s12884-016-0998-5.

Huizink, A. C., Mulder, E. J. H., Robles de Medina, P. G., Visser, G. H. A., & Buitelaar, J. K. (2004). Is pregnancy anxiety a distinctive syndrome? *Early Human Development*. https://pubmed.ncbi.nlm.nih.gov/15324989/.

Hutton, E. K., Reitsma, A. H., & Kaufman, K. (2009). Outcomes associated with planned home and planned hospital births in low-risk women attended by midwives in Ontario, Canada, 2003–2006: A retrospective cohort study. *Birth (Berkeley, Calif)*, 36(3), 180–189.

Jackson, K., Anderson, M., & Marshall, J. E. (2020). Physiology and care during the first stage of labour. In J. Marshall & M. Raynor (Eds.), *Myles textbook for midwives* (17th ed.). London: Elsevier.

Kendig, S., Keats, J. P., Hoffman, C., Kay, L. B., Miller, E. S., Moore Simas, T. A., … Lemieux, L. A. (2017). Consensus bundle on maternal mental health: Perinatal depression and anxiety. *Journal of Obstetric, Gynaecologic and Neonatal Nursing*, 46(2), 272–281. https://pubmed.ncbi.nlm.nih.gov/28190757/.

Kennare, R. M., Keirse, M. J., Tucker, G. R., & Chan, A. C. (2010). Planned home and hospital births in South Australia, 1991–2006: Differences in outcomes. *The Medical Journal of Australia*, 192(2), 76–80.

Khan. L. (2015). *Falling through the gaps: Perinatal mental health and general practice*. Centre for Maternal Health Report.

Khalesi, Z. B., & Bokaie, M. (2018). The association between pregnancy-specific anxiety and preterm birth: A cohort study. *African Health Sciences*, 18(3), 569–575. https://www.ncbi.nlm.nih.gov/pmc/articles/PMC6306999/.

Kirkham. M. (1993). Communication in midwifery. In J. Alexander, V. Levy, & S. Roch (Eds.), *Midwifery practice: A research-based approach*. London: Palgrave.

Lee, S., Ayers, S., & Holden, D. (2016). Risk perception and choice of place of birth in women with high risk pregnancies: A qualitative study. *Midwifery*, 38, 49–54. https://doi.org/10.1016/j.midw.2016.03.008.

Lock, L., & Gibb, H. (2003). The power of place. *Midwifery*, 19(2), 132–139.

Lysell, H., Dahlin, M., Viktorin, A., Ljungberg, E., D'Onofrio, B. M., Dickman, P., & Runeson, B. (2018). Maternal suicide-register based study of all suicides occurring after delivery in Sweden 1974–2009. *PLoS One*, 13(1), e0190133. https://www.ncbi.nlm.nih.gov/pmc/articles/PMC5755764/.

Madeley, A., Williams, V., & McNiven, A. (2019). An interpretative phenomenological study of midwives supporting home birth for women with complex needs. *British Journal of Midwifery*, 27(10), 625–632.

Marks, M. N., Siddle, K., & Warwick, C. (2003). Can we prevent postnatal depression? A randomized controlled trial to assess the effect of continuity of midwifery care on rates of postnatal depression in high-risk women. *The Journal of Maternal, Fetal & Neonatal Medicine*, 13(2), 119–127. https://pubmed.ncbi.nlm.nih.gov/12735413/.

MBRRACE. U. K. (2019). *Saving lives, improving mothers' care. Lessons learned to inform maternity care from the UK and Ireland Confidential Enquiries into Maternal Deaths and Morbidity 2015–17*. Oxford: National Perinatal Epidemiology Unit, University of Oxford.

Meltzer-Brody, S., Howard, L. M., Bergink, V., Vigod, S., Jones, I., Munk-Olsen, T., … Milgrom, J. (2018). Postpartum psychiatric disorders. *Nature Reviews Disease Primers*, 4, 18022. https://pubmed.ncbi.nlm.nih.gov/29695824/.

MIND. (2017). *Anxiety and panic attacks*. https://www.mind.org.uk/information-support/types-of-mental-health-problems/anxiety-and-panic-attacks/about-anxiety/.

Montgomery, E., Pope, C., & Rogers, J. (2015). The re-enactment of childhood sexual abuse in maternity care: A qualitative study. *BMC Pregnancy and Childbirth*, 15, 194.https://doi.org/10.1186/s12884-015-0626-9.

Montgomery v. Lanarkshire Health Board & General Medical Council. UKSC 11, Case Library, 12 King's Bench Walk (online). (2015). Retrieved December 12, 2019 from http://www.12kbw.co.uk/case-library/108/index.html.

Nagle, U., & Farrelly, M. (2018). Women's views and experiences of having their mental health needs considered in the perinatal period. *Midwifery*, 66, 79–87. https://pubmed.ncbi.nlm.nih.gov/30149202/.

National Institute for Health & Care Excellence (NICE). (2014). *Antenatal and postnatal mental health: Clinical management and service guidance. Clinical guideline*. Updated February 2020. https://www.nice.org.uk/guidance/cg192.

National Institute for Health & Care Excellence (NICE). (2017). *Intrapartum care for healthy women and babies* (2nd ed.). London: NICE.

Naylor Smith, J., Taylor, B., Shaw, K., et al. (2018). 'I didn't think you were allowed that, they didn't mention that.' A qualitative study exploring women's perceptions of home birth. *BMC Pregnancy & Childbirth, 18,* 105. https://doi.org/10.1186/s12884-018-1733-1.

NHS England. (2016). *National Maternity Review: Better Births. Improving outcomes of maternity services in England. A five year forward view for maternity care.* London: NHS England.

Nursing & Midwifery Council (NMC) (2018). *The Code Professional standards of practice and behaviour for nurses, midwives and nursing associates.* https://www.nmc.org.uk/globalassets/sitedocuments/nmc-publications/nmc-code.pdf.

Ozlo, I., Leahy-Warren, P., Benyamini, Y., Kazmierczak, M., Karlsdottiir, S. I., Spyridou, A., … Nieuwenhuijze, M. J. (2018). Women's psychological experiences of physiological childbirth: A meta-synthesis. *BMJ Open.* https://bmjopen.bmj.com/content/8/10/e020347.

Public Health England (PHE). (2019). *Guidance: Perinatal mental health.* https://www.gov.uk/government/publications/better-mental-health-jsna-toolkit/4-perinatal-mental-health.

Rayment-Jones, H. T., Murrells, T., & Sandall, J. (2015). An investigation of the relationship between the caseload model of midwifery for socially disadvantaged women and childbirth outcomes using routine data—a retrospective, observational study. *Midwifery, 31*(4), 409–417.

Royal College of Obstetricians and Gynaecologists (RCOG). (2016). *Each baby counts: Key messages from 2015.* London: RCOG.

Royal College of Obstetricians and Gynaecologists (RCOG). (2017). *Maternal mental health-women's voices.* https://www.rcog.org.uk/globalassets/documents/patients/information/maternalmental-healthwomens-voices.pdf.

Renfrew, M., McFadden, A., Bastos, M., Campbell, J., Channon, A., Cheung, N., & Declercq, E. (2014). Midwifery and quality care: Findings from a new evidence-informed framework for maternal and newborn care. *The Lancet, 384*(9948), 1129–1145.

Robertson Blackmore, E., Gustafsson, H., Gilchrist, M., Wyman, C., & O'Connor, T. G. (2016). Pregnancy-related anxiety: Evidence of distinct clinical significance from a prospective longitudinal study. *Journal of Affective Disorders, 197,* 251–258. https://www.ncbi.nlm.nih.gov/pmc/articles/PMC4837058/.

Rowe, H. J., & Fisher, J. R. W. (2010). Development of a universal psycho-educational intervention to prevent common postpartum mental disorders in primiparous women: A multiple method approach. *BMC Public Health, 10,* 499. https://www.ncbi.nlm.nih.gov/pmc/articles/PMC2931475/.

Royal College of Psychiatrists (RCPsyc). (2018). *Mental health in pregnancy*. https://www.rcpsych.ac.uk/mental-health/treatments-and-wellbeing/mental-health-in-pregnancy.

Sandall, J., Soltani, H., Gates, S., Shennan, A., & Devane, D. (2016). Midwife-led continuity models versus other models of care for childbearing women. *Cochrane Database of Systematic Reviews, 4*, CD004667. https://doi.org/10.1002/14651858.CD004667.pub5.

Sandoz, V., Deforges, C., Stuijfzand, S., Epiney, M., Vial, Y., Sekarski, N., … Bickle-Graz, M. (2019). Improving mental health and physiological stress responses in mothers following traumatic childbirth and in their infants: Study protocol for the Swiss TrAumatic biRth Trial (START). *BMJ Open, 9*(12), e032469. https://www.ncbi.nlm.nih.gov/pmc/articles/PMC6955544/.

Simpson, M., & Catling, C. (2016). Understanding psychological traumatic birth experiences: A literature review. *Women & Birth: Journal of Australian College of Midwives, 29*(3), 203–277. https://pubmed.ncbi.nlm.nih.gov/26563636/.

Sinesi, A., Maxwell, M., O'Carroll, R., & Cheyne, H. (2019). Anxiety scales used in pregnancy: Systematic review. *BJPsyc Open, 5*(1), e5. https://www.ncbi.nlm.nih.gov/pmc/articles/PMC6343118/.

The Maternity Transformation Programme. (2020). *Better Births four years on: A review of progress*. NHS England & NHS Improvement. https://www.england.nhs.uk/wp-content/uploads/2020/03/better-births-four-years-on-progress-report.pdf

The Woman's Mental Health Taskforce. (2018). *Final report*. Agenda (Alliance for Women & Girls at Risk). Department of Health & Social Care. https://assets.publishing.service.gov.uk/government/uploads/system/uploads/attachment_data/file/765821/The_Womens_Mental_Health_Taskforce_-_final_report1.pdf.

Viveiros, C. J., & Darling, E. K. (2018). Barriers and facilitators of accessing perinatal mental health services: The perspectives of women receiving continuity of care midwifery. *Midwifery, 65*, 8–15. https://pubmed.ncbi.nlm.nih.gov/30029084/.

World Health Organization (WHO). (2012). *Respectful maternity care: The universal rights of childbearing women*. Washington: White Ribbon Alliance.

Zielinski, R., Ackerson, K., & Low, L. K. (2015). Planned home birth: Benefits, risks, and opportunities. *International Journal of Women's Health, 7*, 361–377.

CHAPTER 8

Men, trans/masculine and non-binary people and midwifery care

Damien W. Riggs, Sally Hines, Carla A. Pfeffer,
Ruth Pearce and Francis Ray White

Growing numbers of men, trans/masculine and non-binary people are considering and undertaking pregnancies (Obedin-Maliver & Makadon, 2016; Tornello & Bos, 2017). In this chapter we use the term "men, trans/masculine and non-binary people" to refer to people who were assigned female at birth but report their identity as, for example, male, man, trans, masculine, trans/masculine, non-binary, genderqueer or agender. Drawing on findings from an original empirical research project on trans pregnancy, this chapter explores men, trans/masculine and non-binary people's experiences with midwives, the views of midwives who provide care to them and the specific challenges that they may face during pregnancy. It also provides recommendations for best practices for midwives working with this diverse population.

The growing body of literature on men, trans/masculine and non-binary people and pregnancy suggests that pregnancy, birthing and infant feeding can be a distressing experience for some (Obedin-Maliver & Makadon, 2016). Research also shows that the pre-conception period can be a particularly challenging and lonely time (Ellis, Wojnar, & Pettinato, 2014). This may be particularly so given that the pre-conception period may involve pausing testosterone administration, and due to the fact that other people commonly view pregnancy, birth and chestfeeding as inherently feminine actions. By contrast, some men, trans/masculine and non-binary people experience pregnancy, birth and chestfeeding as affirming: each demonstrates that the body has purpose and utility in terms of the aim of having and sustaining the life of a child (MacDonald et al., 2016). Again, this is especially true when people are affirmed as masculine or non-gendered in their role as a gestational parent, father or dad by others (including health care professionals).

To date, there has been very little published literature on midwives and men, trans/masculine and non-binary people. One Swedish study found that midwives feel they lack knowledge about men, trans/masculine and non-binary people and pregnancy, but that they want to be inclusive even if they are not sure how (Johansson, Wirén, Ssempasa, & Wells, 2020). Midwives in this study recognised the importance of continuity of care to ensure that men, trans/masculine and non-binary people do not have to repeatedly explain themselves. A study of midwives in the United States found that for trans men who were midwives, some experienced stigma, and others felt they were pressured by colleagues and administrators not to disclose their gender history to other staff or patients (Kantrowitz-Gordon, Ellis, & McFarlane, 2014). While in some contexts there has a been a shift away from the language of 'mothers' and 'women' within midwifery associations to be more inclusive of all genders (i.e. instead using 'pregnant people'), there has been considerable opposition to this by some midwives and midwife organisations (Reis, 2020). Finally, some research has suggested that the push towards chestfeeding by midwives can be experienced as distressing by some men, trans/masculine and non-binary people (MacDonald et al., 2016).

In our own research, in which we interviewed 51 men, trans/masculine and non-binary people living in the United States, Canada, the United Kingdom, Australia, Bulgaria and Germany, many of our participants spoke about experiences with midwives. For some of our participants, their experiences with midwives were positive. Positive experiences included midwives consistently asking for consent to touch men, trans/masculine and non-binary people's bodies; amending documentation (including on paper and electronically) to ensure gender is correctly recorded; and advocating for participants, for example, through going out of their way to ensure that other staff used correct names and pronouns. Some participants felt especially supported by midwives who disclosed that they had trans/masculine or non-binary family members, and other participants commented on how positive it was to be supported by midwives who are men.

Some of our participants, however, had negative experiences with midwives. Examples of negative experiences included midwives dismissing the importance of using the correct terminology for their body parts; midwives equating men, trans/masculine and non-binary people's experiences of birth with those of cisgender (i.e. non-transgender) women; and midwives repeatedly misgendering (e.g. using the wrong name or pronouns) men, trans/masculine and non-binary people despite being corrected on multiple occasions. Importantly, our participants did not expect midwives to be perfect; rather, they expected that midwives would do their best to work with them to understand their specific needs.

In our study, we also interviewed a small number of midwives who had experience working with men, trans/masculine and non-binary people and pregnancy, including two midwives who were themselves transgender.

These participants noted a number of challenges to the full inclusion of men, trans/masculine and non-binary people within midwifery services. These included the lack of training provided about working with men, trans/masculine and non-binary people; both a lack of awareness about trans-specific pregnancy needs and an over-focus on men, trans/masculine and non-binary people's gender at the expense of focussing on their pregnancy; the expectation placed upon transgender midwives to educate other people, often without compensation; a lack of medical knowledge about postpartum care for men, trans/masculine and non-binary people, particularly in regard to chestfeeding and recommencing hormone therapies; and animosity within the profession towards the inclusion of men, trans/masculine and non-binary people.

Both our research and that of others suggest a number of key recommendations for further developing best practice approaches for supporting men, trans/masculine and non-binary people within midwifery services:

1. Ask patients about the pronouns, names and terminology they use to describe themselves and their bodies. Collate this information and ensure that all relevant staff are aware. It should not be the work of men, trans/masculine and non-binary people to continually educate staff.

2. Provide training opportunities and stay engaged with the latest literature. Research on men, trans/masculine and non-binary people is a fast-moving field requiring continuous monitoring and engagement.

3. Ensure high-quality continuity of care so that men, trans/masculine and non-binary people are able to work with individual care providers and care teams intimately familiar with them and their specific case.

4. Avoid simplistically comparing experiences. While some of the physical aspects of birthing may be shared, others will be specific or unique for men, trans/masculine and non-binary people due to both their own experiences of sex/gender and those of people around them.

5. Be aware that for some (but not all) men, trans/masculine and non-binary people, pregnancy and birthing may be specifically distressing, and engage in practices that attempt to minimise distress, such as explicitly negotiating consent regarding touch, delivery procedures and using patient-led language.

6. Advocate for systemic change, even in the face of opposition. This includes but is not limited to resource allocation towards incorporating inclusive and diverse imagery and language (e.g. 'pregnant person' or 'pregnant people') in offices, on forms, in educational and training materials, in electronic medical records and in interactions with care recipients.

7. Recognise that chestfeeding may not be possible for some men, trans/masculine and non-binary people, and for other people it may be distressing. Further, some men, trans/masculine and non-binary people

may need specific support to encourage skills for chestfeeding if that is their desire (i.e. if they have already had chest surgery); such support must also be trans-informed and inclusive.

8. Advocate for and engage in research that seeks to better understand the specific social and medical needs of men, trans/masculine and non-binary people, specifically in terms of best practices regarding recommencement of hormone therapies.

In conclusion, for many men, trans/masculine and non-binary people, pregnancy and birth can be a positive experience, but this is dependent on how other people (including health care providers) respond, specifically in terms of using inclusive language. For some men, trans/masculine and non-binary people, pregnancy and birth may be distressing. However, this can be minimised by the use of inclusive language and respect for bodily autonomy. As the numbers of men, trans/masculine and non-binary people becoming gestational parents continue to grow, it is important that midwives continue to grow alongside this population: growing their skills, understandings and openness to supporting men, trans/masculine and non-binary people.

Acknowledgments

Damien W. Riggs, College of Education, Psychology and Social Work, Flinders University. Carla A. Pfeffer, Department of Sociology, University of South Carolina. Sally Hines, Department of Sociological Studies, University of Sheffield. Ruth Pearce, Trans Learning Partnership and School of Sociology and Social Policy, University of Leeds. Francis Ray White, School of Social Sciences, Westminster University.

Funded by the Economic and Social Research Council, ES/N019067/1.

References

Ellis, S. A., Wojnar, D. M., & Pettinato, M. (2014). Conception, pregnancy, and birth experiences of male and gender variant gestational parents: It's how we could have a family. *Journal of Midwifery & Women's Health*, 60(1), 62–69.

Johansson, M., Wirén, A. A., Ssempasa, D., & Wells, M. (2020). A qualitative study of midwives' challenges to support transmen during childbirth: A short report. *The European Journal of Midwifery*.

Kantrowitz-Gordon, I., Ellis, S. A., & McFarlane, A. (2014). Men in midwifery: A national survey. *Journal of Midwifery & Women's Health*, 59(5), 516–522.

MacDonald, T., Noel-Weiss, J., West, D., Walks, M., Biener, M., Kibbe, A., & Myler, E. (2016). Transmasculine individuals' experiences with lactation, chestfeeding, and gender identity: A qualitative study. *BMC Pregnancy and Childbirth*, 16(1), 1–17.

Obedin-Maliver, J., & Makadon, H. J. (2016). Transgender men and pregnancy. *Obstetric Medicine*, 9(1), 4–8.

Reis, E. (2020). Midwives and pregnant men: Labouring toward ethical care in the United States. *Canadian Medical Association Journal*, 192, 169–170.

Tornello, S. L., & Bos, H. (2017). Parenting intentions among transgender individuals. *LGBT Health*, 4(2), 115–120.

Questions for reflection

1. What are three concrete steps you can take to work towards ensuring that the forms, artwork, pamphlets and educational materials at your midwifery worksite are inclusive of trans and gender non-binary parents and families?

2. What are three concrete steps you can take with your colleagues to ensure that the midwifery staff (clerical, administrative and medical providers) are working towards trans and gender non-binary inclusive, ethical and culturally competent patient interactions and care?

3. What are three concrete steps you can take to engage in outreach to your professional midwifery organisation(s) to ensure that they are inclusive and advocating on behalf of trans and gender non-binary people who are pregnant?

Further reading and resources

Fischer, O. J. (2020). Non-binary reproduction: Stories of conception, pregnancy, and birth. *International Journal of Transgender Health*.

Hoffkling, A., Obedin-Maliver, J., & Sevelius, J. (2017). From erasure to opportunity: A qualitative study of the experiences of transgender men around pregnancy and recommendations for providers. *BMC Pregnancy and Childbirth*, 17.

MacDonald, T. (2016). *Where's the mother? Stories from a transgender dad*. Toronto: Trans Canada Press.

Midwives Alliance of North America. (2015). *Position statement on gender inclusive language*. https://mana.org/healthcare-policy/position-statement-on-gender-inclusive-language.

Moseson, H., Zazanis, N., Goldberg, E., Fix, L., Durden, M., Stoeffler, A., Hastings, J., … Obedin-Maliver, J. (2020). The imperative for transgender and gender nonbinary inclusion. *Obstetrics & Gynecology*, 135(5), 1059–1068.

Silver, A. J. (2019). Birth beyond the binary. *AIMS Journal*, 31(2). https://www.aims.org.uk/journal/item/non-binary-birth.

CHAPTER 9

Exploration of extraneous factors that may contribute to the development of perinatal mental illness

Michelle Anderson

There are many factors that can contribute to the development of perinatal mental illness (PMI). This final chapter aims to explore how some of the facets of modern-day life may have an impact on pregnancy and mental health.

Part 1: The global pandemic

COVID-19

COVID-19 precipitated a tsunami of change which had implications for both physical and psychological health. The UK national lockdown in March 2020 and subsequent municipal lockdowns and national lockdowns placed unprecedented restrictions on a free-willed society. The balance between controlling the spread of COVID-19 and reducing its economic, physical and mental health impact felt, at times, much like teetering on a cliff edge. Humanity grappled with a virus that relied on a lack of social compliance. Much of the population wrestled with their social conscience by conforming to socially restrictive measures (and understanding the importance of them) while recognising that a significant proportion of society were left feeling isolated and alone. Thus the effects of COVID-19 are far reaching and socially complex, as with all pandemics.

The restrictive social measures implemented to delay the spread of COVID-19 are themselves key risk factors for deteriorating mental health in the general population (Anderson, 2020). Factors such as social disconnection, lack of meaning (purpose) and financial stress all contribute to poor mental health (Holmes et al., 2020) and the uncertainty of living through a pandemic and making life-changing alterations is likely to increase anxiety levels in much of the population (Kroenke, Spitzer, Williams, Monahan, & Lowe, 2007).

COVID-19 caused increased anxiety for many pregnant women (Royal College of Midwives (RCM), 2020a, 2020b), especially during the initial first wave of infections, as little was known about the effects of COVID-19 in pregnancy. Many pregnant women had other stressors to consider aside from being pregnant, such as financial implications, loss of employment and childcare. In fact, one study found that pregnant women were less concerned about their own health and more concerned about the health of older relatives, their own children and, finally, the pregnancy (Corbett, Milne, Hehir, Lindow, & O'Connell, 2020). However, another study reported that the number of women with high anxiety levels doubled during the pandemic with concerns about how COVID-19 might affect their babies. Anxiety included fears about foetal abnormalities, foetal growth restriction and pre-term birth (Mappa, Distefano, & Rizzo, 2020).

Measures put in place by UK hospitals to reduce the spread of the virus may have added to anxiety in pregnant women. Women were told that partners could not accompany them during antenatal and scan appointments, and visits to antenatal and postnatal wards were restricted. This resulted in women receiving less support from partners and family members prior to or post birth.

My own research into how pregnant women have been affected psychologically by COVID-19 (at the time of writing, data collection is still ongoing) has facilitated meaningful discussions with women. The following statements are from an interim analysis of a small number of women who participated in semi-structured interviews on COVID-19 and pregnancy:

+   'I felt alone during scan and ward admissions'
+   'Hearing on the news that people were dying every day scared me'
+   'I was worried my partner wouldn't be able to come to labour ward with me'
+   'Hearing (in the media) that black, Asian and minority ethnic (BAME) women might be more at risk really scared me'
+   'I felt alone'
+   'I didn't consider myself to be an anxious person, but I have felt really anxious'
+   'My partner felt detached'

These disclosures give some insight into how women felt during the pandemic. 'Feeling alone' appeared to be a common theme, suggesting that women may have felt isolated during the pandemic, even if they lived with a supportive partner. It could be suggested that the subjective experience of fear itself could magnify feelings of isolation, especially if there is a high level of uncertainty surrounding a given situation, as was the case during the pandemic.

The *Babies in Lockdown* report (2020) analysed 5474 respondents who completed an online survey investigating the impact of COVID-19 on babies and parents across the UK (Parent-Infant Foundation, 2020). Findings included the following:

+ Many families with lower incomes and BAME communities were hit harder by the COVID-19 pandemic.
+ Almost 7 in 10 parents (68%) felt the changes brought about by COVID-19 were affecting their unborn baby, baby or young child.
+ Almost 87% of parents were more anxious as a result of COVID-19 and lockdown.
+ 68% of respondents said their ability to cope with their pregnancy or baby has been impacted by COVID-19, and this figure was highest for Asian/Asian British respondents.
+ Fewer Asian/Asian British and black/black British respondents felt they had the information they needed during pregnancy or after birth compared with white respondents.
+ Over one-third (34%) of those who gave birth during lockdown stated that care at birth was not as planned.
+ 28% of respondents felt they did not receive the breastfeeding support they required.

Our clinical understanding of COVID-19 has increased significantly. We now know that most women who experience COVID-19 develop only mild symptoms and that vertical transmission is uncommon and not affected by mode of birth (Royal College of Obstetricians and Gynaecologists (RCOG), 2020). However, maternal COVID-19 is associated with approximately three times greater risk of pre-term birth and caesarean section birth (RCOG, 2020).

It is also worth noting that there are a number of risk factors which appear to be associated with severe COVID-19 and hospital admission:

+ BAME background
+ Being overweight (body mass index (BMI) $25-29\,kg/m^2$) or obese (BMI $30\,kg/m^2$ or more)
+ Pre-pregnancy co-morbidity, such as pre-existing diabetes and chronic hypertension
+ Maternal age 35 years or older
+ Living in areas or households of increased socioeconomic deprivation
+ Infection with COVID-19 more common if occupation increases exposure frequency, such as working in health care or other public facing professions (RCOG, 2020).

It is especially important to acknowledge the impact of the pandemic on BAME women. The UK Obstetric Surveillance System (UKOSS) report (2020) found that more than half of pregnant women admitted to the hospital with SARS-CoV-2 infection in pregnancy were from black or other ethnic minority groups. It is perhaps worth noting that increased hospital admissions have been seen for ethnic minority groups in the non-pregnant population, too. Reasons for this may include social behaviours, health behaviours, co-morbidities and potentially genetic influences (Knight et al., 2020). However, further research is needed to investigate these assumptions. In the context of PMI, BAME women may be at risk of increased anxiety relating to COVID-19 and pregnancy. Therefore midwives should do their best to offer reassurance where possible.

Additional factors exacerbated by the pandemic

Domestic abuse

It is well documented that domestic abuse increases during pregnancy (Finnbogadottir & Karin-Dykes, 2016; see Chapter 4 for further details). Lockdown may have had severe consequences for women in already abusive relationships or may have been a trigger for others in the initiation of domestic abuse. During lockdown, domestic abuse charities reported higher than usual calls to help-lines and online services (RCM, 2020a, 2020b). The charity Refuge reported a 700% increase in calls over a single day during lockdown and a 25% increase in calls from perpetrators seeking to change their behaviour (Townsend, 2020). This makes for harrowing reading and perhaps demonstrates the difficult and dangerous situations many women faced during the lockdown period.

The feeling of being alone

Although many pregnant women enjoy supportive relationships with their partners, some women may rely on support from outside of the home. Other women may not have partners at all, perhaps after going through a relationship breakdown or planning and choosing to go though pregnancy independently. There is, of course, nothing nicer than meeting up with a group of friends and putting the world to rights. This changed during lockdown.

A qualitative study investigating the effects of isolation and mood in pregnant women in the second and third trimester found an interesting dichotomy. Although many women reported that their relationships with their partners did not deteriorate during lockdown and many women enjoyed 'the break from life's fast pace', nearly half of women reported low mood due to loneliness and missing contact with family and friends (Milne, Corbett, Hehir, & Lindow, 2020).

Human beings are social by nature, and during the pandemic, loneliness increased globally throughout the general population (Groarke et al., 2020). Risk factors for loneliness include having a previous mental health condition, being female and having a low income (Groarke et al., 2020). It is difficult to know if pregnancy may be a protective factor for some against loneliness, as pregnancy itself gives women a purpose and focus, which could be seen as important in the face of uncertainty.

Stress

Research has shown that during the pandemic, women were more likely to take responsibility for childcare, including home schooling while trying to juggle working from home (Savage, 2020). This has been termed by some as the 'caregiver burden', and COVID-19 exacerbated caregiving responsibilities, which tend to fall to women (Conner et al., 2020). The pandemic has highlighted that gender inequality remains and that disproportionate expectations are placed on women when societal structures become skewed.

In short, we do not yet know the long-term affects of COVID-19 both on physical and mental health, but it is without doubt that there will be long-term implications. Although we cannot predict whether subsequent pandemics will take place (although it is possible in our lifetime), we need to ensure that we learn from the impact of COVID-19 and that resources are in place to support women and their families in the event of subsequent public health calamities.

Part 2: Digital and social media

Over the past few decades there has been a rapid, epochal shift from industry to information technology. This transition has transformed how we live our lives, especially since the emergence of the World Wide Web. We have information at our fingertips, we can shop and socialise online, we can connect with fellow human beings in a way that we have never been able to before – the list is endless! Technology and the way we use it is firmly embedded within modern-day existence and, through the very nature of adaptation, human behaviour has changed to embrace technological advancement. Although there are many benefits to technology, how we use it can have consequences. Yamamoto and Ananou (2015) posit the negative cognitive, social, emotional and ethical implications of digital use, pointing out the importance of using technology in a positive way to minimise the negative impact on humans. Exploring the negative impact of digital use is crucial if we are to understand it in the context of mental health.

There is much debate on whether digital technology affects mental health (Haidt & Allen, 2020). However, correlataional data suggest that a rise in mental health disorders over the past few decades appear to correspond with increased screen-based activity (Hrafnkeldottir et al., 2018), and this is particularly so in adolescents (Haidt & Allen, 2020). Type of screen time use may vary, but another factor potentially contributing to the rise in mental health disorders is social media. A number of studies have reported that increased social media and multi-platform use is associated with anxiety and depression (Becker, Alzahabi, & Hopwood, 2013; Vannucci, Flannery, & Ohannessinn, 2017).

Negative aspects of social media can include the following:

- Feeling a sense of inadequacy (e.g. comparing life experiences to others on social media).
- Fear of missing out, which social media can exacerbate and cause frequent checking for updates on social media platforms.
- Isolation: High use of social media may increase feelings of loneliness.
- Cyberbullying: Social media platforms can help to facilitate bullying behaviour by making it easier to leave comments anonymously.
- Self-absorption: Constantly sharing 'selfies' and posting updates can create an unhealthy self-centredness and detachment from real life connections (Robinson & Smith, 2020).

Women are disproportionally affected by anxiety (Remes, Brayne, Van Der Linde, & Lafortune, 2016). The reason for this is multi-factorial, but in the context of social media, anxiety has been linked to preoccupation with body image, low self-esteem, mood changes and feeling less physically attractive (Mills, Musto, Williams, & Tiggemann, 2018). This is probably because women are more likely to maintain and manage their social profiles (Perloff, 2014) and upload photos to social media more frequently than men (Mills et al., 2018). This might be in an attempt to conform to stereotypical perceptions of (Western) beauty, which becomes an unrealistic endeavour when trying to compete with filters and Photoshop. No doubt some women of childbearing age will fall into this category and this may set the precedence for social media use during pregnancy.

During pregnancy, digital and social media may take on a different function. Pregnant women may use digital media for a variety of reasons, such as information seeking and information sharing (Oviatt & Reich, 2019). In fact, one of the benefits of digital and social media is being able to connect with others in a positive way, such as to build support networks and participate in online group discussions. However, information received from media platforms can sometimes be inaccurate (Harpel, 2018) and users can sometimes become burdened by too much choice (Oviatt & Reich, 2019).

A risk factor for anxiety may be exposure to false representations of pregnancy and motherhood on social media platforms. Images posted of the 'perfect' pregnancy and birth may give rise to feelings of inadequacy in some women. One study found that 'over-sharing' of idealistic family images may also lead to anxiety amongst parents and that 'mummy blogging' may be contributing to depression (Priory Group, 2020). This might be especially true for women with complex social issues or those women with existing mental health conditions.

It is worth considering the benefits associated with digital media use alongside the negatives. As discussed, digital and social media platforms can prove effective in providing information about pregnancy, birth and parenting. However, overuse of media platforms or accessing information from less reputable sources may cause psychological distress and increase the risk of anxiety and depression. Social media use may also differ cross-culturally, and more research is needed to properly evaluate the positive and negative impact of social media on pregnant women and mothers.

References

Anderson. M. (2020). Covid-19: A discussion on pregnancy, birth and psychological well-being. *MIDIRS Midwifery Digest*, 30(3), 344–347.

Becker, M. W., Alzahabi, R., & Hopwood, C. J. (2013). Media multitasking is associated with symptoms of depression and social anxiety. *Cyber Psychology, Behaviour & Social Networking*, 16(2), 132–135. https://pubmed.ncbi.nlm.nih.gov/23126438/.

Conner, J., Madhavan, S., Mokashi, M., Amanuel, H., Johnson, N. R., Pace, L. E., & Bartz, D. (2020). Health risks and outcomes that disproportionately affect women during the Covid-19 pandemic: A review. *Society of Scientific Medicine*, 266, 113364. https://www.ncbi.nlm.nih.gov/pmc/articles/PMC7487147/.

Corbett, G. A., Milne, S. J., Hehir, M. P., Lindow, S. W., & O'Connell, M. P. (2020). Health anxiety and behavioural changes of pregnant women during the COVID-19 pandemic. *European Journal of Obstetrics & Gynaecology and Reproductive Health*, 249, 96–97. https://www.ncbi.nlm.nih.gov/pmc/articles/PMC7194619/.

Finnbogadottir, H., & Karin-Dykes, A. (2016). Increasing prevalence and incidence of domestic violence during the pregnancy and one and a half year postpartum, as well as risk factors: A longitudinal cohort study in southern Sweden. *BMC Pregnancy & Childbirth*. https://link.springer.com/article/10.1186/s12884-016-1122-6.

Groarke, J. M., Berry, E., Graham-Wisener, L., Mckenna-Plumley, P. E., McGlinchey, E., & Armour, C. (2020). Loneliness in the UK during the COVID-19 pandemic: Cross-sectional results from the COVID-19 Psychological Wellbeing Study. *PLoS One*, 15(9), e0239698. https://www.ncbi.nlm.nih.gov/pmc/articles/PMC7513993/.

Haidt, J., & Allen, N. (2020). Scrutinizing the effects of digital technology on mental health. *Nature*. https://www.nature.com/articles/d41586-020-00296-x.

Harpel. T. (2018). Pregnant women sharing pregnancy-related information on Facebook: Web-based survey study. *Journal of Medical Internet Research*, 20(3), e115. https://www.ncbi.nlm.nih.gov/pmc/articles/PMC5887042/.

Holmes, E. A., O'Connor, R. C., Perry, H. V., Tracey, I., Wessely, S., Arseneault, L., … Bullmore, E. (2020). Multi-disciplinary research priorities for the Covid-19 pandemic: A call for action for mental health science. *Lancet Psychiatry*, 7, 547–560.

Hrafnkeldottir, S. M., Brychta, R. J., Rognvaldsdottir, V., Gestsdottir, S., Johannsson, E., Guomundsdottir, S. L., & Arngrimsson, S. A. (2018). Less screen time and more frequent vigorous physical activity is associated with lower risk of reporting negative mental health symptoms among Icelandic adolescents. *PLoS One*, 13(4), e0196286. https://www.ncbi.nlm.nih.gov/pmc/articles/PMC5919516/.

Knight, M., Bunch, K., Vousden, N., Morris, E., Simpson, N., Gale, C., … Kurinczuk, J. J. (2020). Characteristics and outcomes of pregnant women admitted to hospital with confirmed SARS-CoV-2 infection in UK: National population based cohort study. *The British Medical Journal*. https://doi.org/10.1136/bmj.m2107.

Kroenke, K., Spitzer, R. I., Williams, J. B. W., Monahan, P. O., & Lowe, B. (2007). Anxiety disorders in primary care: Prevalence, impairment, co morbidity, and detection. *Annals of Internal Medicine*, 146(5), 317–325.

Mappa, I., Distefano, F. A., & Rizzo, G. (2020). Effects of coronavirus 19 pandemic on maternal anxiety during pregnancy: A prospective observational study. *Journal of Perinatal Medicine*, 48(6), 545–550. https://pubmed.ncbi.nlm.nih.gov/32598320/.

Mills, J. S., Musto, S., Williams, L., & Tiggemann, M. (2018). "Selfie" harm: Effects on mood and body image in young women. *Body Image*, 27, 86–92. https://www.sciencedirect.com/science/article/pii/S1740144517305326?via%3Dihub.

Milne, S. J., Corbett, G. A., Hehir, M. P., & Lindow, S. W. (2020). Effects of isolation on mood and relationships in pregnant women during the covid-19 pandemic. *European Journal of Obstetrics & Gynaecology and Reproductive Health*, 252, 610–611. https://www.ncbi.nlm.nih.gov/pmc/articles/PMC7278652/.

Oviatt, J. R., & Reich, S. M. (2019). Pregnancy posting: Exploring characteristics of social media posts around pregnancy and user engagement. *mHealth*, 5, 46. https://www.ncbi.nlm.nih.gov/pmc/articles/PMC6851430/.

Parent-Infant Foundation. (2020). *Babies in lockdown: Listening to parents to build back better*. Best Beginnings, Home-Start UK, and the Parent-Infant Foundation.

Perloff. R. M. (2014). Social media effects on young women's body image concerns: Theoretical perspectives and an agenda for research. *Sex Roles, 71,* 363–377. https://doi.org/10.1007/s11199-014-0384-6.

Priory Group. (2020). *Is social media fuelling anxiety and depression among parents?* https://www.priorygroup.com/blog/is-social-media-fuelling-anxiety-and-depression-among-parents

Remes, O., Brayne, C., Van Der Linde, R., & Lafortune, L. (2016). A systematic review of reviews on the prevalence of anxiety disorders in adult populations. *Brain & Behaviour, 6*(7), e00497. https://www.ncbi.nlm.nih.gov/pmc/articles/PMC4951626/.

Robinson, L., & Smith, M. (2020). *Social media & mental health.* HelpGuide. https://www.helpguide.org/articles/mental-health/social-media-and-mental-health.htm.

Royal College of Midwives (RCM). (2020a). *RCM clinical guidance briefing perinatal mental health care during Covid-19.* https://www.rcm.org.uk/media/3859/rcm-clinical-guidance-briefing-no-10-perinatal-mental-health-care.pdf.

Royal College of Midwives (RCM). (2020b). *Identifying, caring for and supporting women at risk of/victims of domestic abuse during COVID-19.* Version 1. https://www.rcm.org.uk/media/4067/identifying-caring-for-and-supporting-women-at-risk-of_victims-of-domestic-abuse-during-covid-19-v1__13052020final.pdf.

Royal College of Obstetricians and Gynaecologists (RCOG). (2020). Coronavirus (Covid-19) infection in pregnancy. Information for healthcare professionals. Version 12. https://www.rcog.org.uk/en/guidelines-research-services/guidelines/coronavirus-pregnancy/.

Savage, M. (2020). As working mums perform more childcare and face increased job insecurity, there are fears Covid-19 has undone decades of advancement. But could the pandemic be a catalyst for progress? https://www.bbc.com/worklife/article/20200630-how-covid-19-is-changing-womens-lives.

Townsend, M. (2020). Revealed: Surge in domestic violence during COVID-19 crisis. *The Observer.* Retrieved May 22, 2020 from https://www.theguardian.com/society/2020/apr/12/domestic-violence-surges-seven-hundred-per-cent-uk-coronavirus.

Vannucci, A., Flannery, K. M., & Ohannessinn, C. M. (2017). Social media use and anxiety in emerging adults. *Journal of Affective Disorders, 207,* 163–166. https://pubmed.ncbi.nlm.nih.gov/27723539/.

Yamamoto, J., & Ananou, S. (2015). *Humanity in the digital age: Cognitive, social, emotional, and ethical implications.* Contemporary Educational Technology. https://files.eric.ed.gov/fulltext/EJ1105609.pdf.

Appendix

Michelle Anderson

Useful websites/resources

General resources

Fatherhood Institute: www.fatherhoodinstitute.org

Maternal Mental Health Alliance: https://maternalmentalhealthalliance.org/resource-hub

MIND: www.mind.org.uk

National Childbirth Trust: https://www.nct.org.uk

National Institute for Health and Care Excellence (UK): https://www.nice.org.uk

NHS Digital: https://www.digital.nhs.uk

Perinatal Illness UK: https://www.chimat.org.uk

Perinatal Mental Health Toolkit by the Royal College of General Practitioners: https://www.rcgp.org.uk/clinical-and-research/resources/toolkits/perinatal-mental-health-toolkit.aspx

Perinatal Mental Health: https://fingertips.phe.org.uk/profile-group/mental-health/profile/perinatal-mental-health

Royal College of Psychiatrists (UK): https://www.rcpsych.ac.uk

The International Marcé Society for Perinatal Mental Health: https://marcesociety.com

Trans Pregnancy: https://transpregnancy.leeds.ac.uk/about/

Resources for specific mental health issues

Anxiety & depression

MIND: https://www.mind.org.uk/search-results?q=perinatal%20mental%20health

NHS Choices: Postnatal depression: www.nhs.uk/conditions/postnatal depression/Pages/Introduction.aspx

Pandas Foundation: Pre and postnatal depression advice and support: https://www.pandasfoundation.org.uk

PND & Me: Raising awareness of perinatal mental health: https://www.pndandme.co.uk

Royal College of Psychiatrists: Postnatal depression – key facts: https://www.rcpsych.ac.uk/mental-health/problems-disorders/postnatal-depression-key-facts

Tommy's: Postnatal depression (PND): https://www.tommys.org/pregnancy-information/im-pregnant/mental-wellbeing/specific-mental-health-conditions/postnatal-depression-pnd

Association for Postnatal Illness: https://www.apni.org/

ADHD

ADHD UK: https://www.adhduk.co.uk/

Bipolar

Action on Postpartum Psychosis: https://www.app-network.org

Association for Postnatal Illness: https://www.apni.org

Bipolar UK: Women and Bipolar: https://www.bipolaruk.org/Pages/FAQs/Category/women-and-bipolar

Eating disorders

For patients and professionals, who require specific information about pregnancy:

http://www.eatingdisordersandpregnancy.co.uk/

For individuals suffering with EDs:

https://www.beateatingdisorders.org.uk/

https://www.caraline.com/

https://firststepsed.co.uk/

https://www.therecoveryclub.org/resources

https://www.anorexiabulimiacare.org.uk/

https://www.recoverywarriors.com/

For parents of people who suffer from EDs:

https://www.feast-ed.org/

OCD

https://maternalocd.org/

https://www.rcpsych.ac.uk/mental-health/problems-disorders/perinatal-ocd

Personality disorders

https://www.rcpsych.ac.uk/mental-health/problems-disorders/
    personality-disorder
http://personalitydisorder.org.uk/
https://www.rethink.org/advice-and-information/about-mental-illness/
    learn-more-about-conditions/borderline-personality-disorder/
https://www.cope.org.au/wp-content/uploads/2017/11/BPD-in-
    Perinatal-Period_Consumer-Fact-Sheet.pdf – this is a useful printable
    factsheet about BPD and pregnancy (however, the source is Australian,
    and information about accessing help is *not* relevant to the UK)

PTSD

https://www.ptsduk.org/
https://www.ptsduk.org/what-is-ptsd/post-natal-ptsd/
https://www.birthtraumaassociation.org.uk/

Schizophrenia

https://www.nhs.uk/conditions/Schizophrenia/
https://livingwithschizophreniauk.org/

INDEX

Page numbers followed by *b* indicates boxes, *f* indicates figures and *t* indicates tables.